IMMUNE POWER

**PREVENTION'S LIBRARY
OF MEDICAL CARE AND NATURAL HEALING**™

IMMUNE POWER

by the Editors of Prevention®
Magazine Health Books

 Rodale Press, Emmaus, Pennsylvania

Printed in the United States of America on acid-free paper containing a high percentage of recycled fiber.

Library of Congress Cataloging-in-Publication Data

Immune power.

(Prevention's library of medical care and natural healing)
Includes index.
1. Immunity—Popular works.   I. Prevention (Emmaus, Pa.)   II. Series.
QR185.3.I44   1989   616.07'9   88-26441
ISBN 0-87857-787-4   hardcover

2 4 6 8 10 9 7 5 3 1   hardcover

NOTICE

PREVENTION'S LIBRARY OF MEDICAL CARE AND NATURAL HEALING™

Series Editor: Carol Keough

Immune Power **Editors:** William Gottlieb, Debora Tkac, John Feltman, Mark Bricklin

Writing Contributions

Kim Anderson
  Fitness and Sports, Outdoors, Smallpox, Travel, Weather, 40 Worst Infections

Don Barone
  Children, Self-Care for Everyday Infections

Alice Feinstein
  Heredity, How Your Immune System Works, Medical Frontiers, Your Mind and Your Immune System, Xenobiotic Infections

Marcia Holman
  Detecting Infection, Nutrition and Immunity

Judith Lin
  Drugs and the Immune System, Home, Infection Fighting at the CDC, Medications, Pets, Smoking

Ellen Michaud
  Immunity and Cancer

Russell Wild
  Emergency Infections, Food, Hospitals, Plague, Regional Infections, Sex

CONTENTS

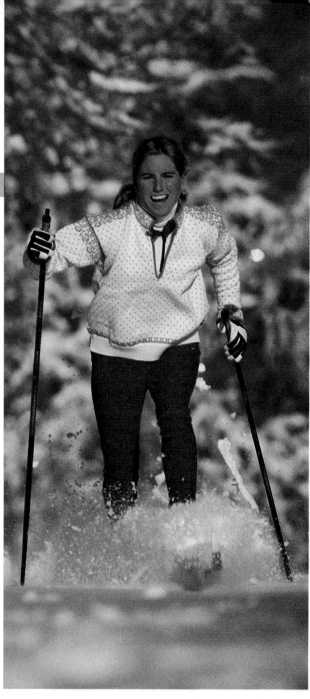

Staying active, staying well, see pp. 26–27.

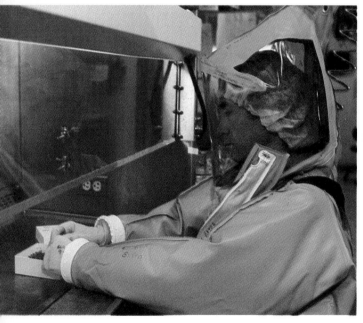

Germ warfare in action, see p. 67.

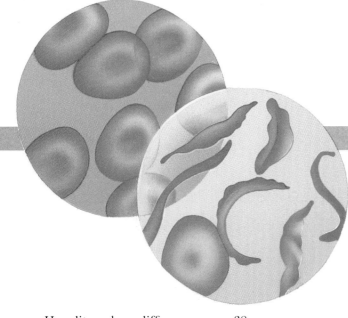

Heredity makes a difference, see p. 38.

Heredity makes a difference, see p. 38.

O

Infection protection starts early, see p. 12.

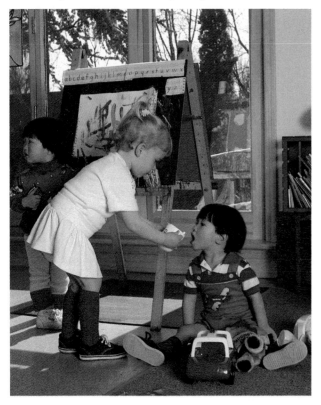

R

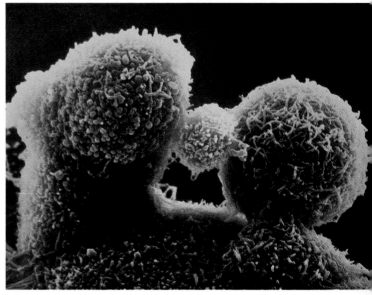

Beating the cancer cell, see pp. 62–63.

Beating the cancer cell, see pp. 62–63.

T

PREFACE THE PATH TO PROTECTION

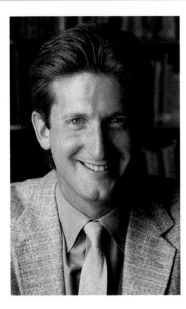

When the writers here at Prevention Magazine Health Books were working on *Immune Power* there was a reference book around the office that never managed to stay on one person's shelf for long. It contained photographs, taken with the help of an electron microscope, of the cellular components of the immune system. There was something compelling and awesome—even frightening—about those pictures, like looking into a mirror and seeing the skeleton under your skin.

Here were the tiny knights of their blood, the miniature guardians of their lives—and these cells looked and acted like a cross between a pit bull and a slug. Twenty tentacles looped out from a lump of a body to snare and strangle a hapless bit of bacteria. So-called killer cells stuck invading microbes with dozens of deadly spikes, while another bunch of definitely uncouth defenders cleaned up by dining on the remains. The writers didn't know whether to cringe or cheer, whether they were still health writers or had somehow been transformed into war correspondents—and the gruesome battles they had to cover were in their own bodies!

But over the months of putting together this book, of reading the scientific studies and interviewing the experts—of finding out, for you, the best ways to keep the immune system at its most powerful and effective—they came to understand and admire the army within.

An army so efficient that its "boot camp"—the bone marrow—turns out over a million new soldiers every second.

An army so resourceful that it uses the genetic code of the body to manufacture a unique weapon against each and every disease entity it has to battle.

An army so central to our health that its total defeat at the hands of an insidious virus is the story of the decade, the sad specter of AIDS.

And they learned that this army depends on you. It's nourished by the food you eat and strengthened by the exercise you get. Your thoughts and feelings are a kind of weather: In the sunshine of confidence and love, the army is on the march, but it's slowed by the cold rain of anger and despair. And the soldiers in this army are smart enough to appreciate when your doctor scouts for disease or enlists the reinforcements of medication.

This book, then, is your field manual, a guide to the military science of martialing your immune army—it tells you everything you need to know to protect yourself and your family from surrendering to disease.

William Gottlieb

William Gottlieb
Editorial Director, Prevention® Magazine Health Books

CHILDREN

There's no sound. Your house is completely dark, except for the yellow glow emanating from the Big Bird nightlight in the bathroom. You're just about to drift into serious sleep. Then it happens.

"Mommy . . . . Daddy . . . I don't feel good!"

It's like the sound of squealing brakes in the middle of the night. You lie there semi-awake, waiting for the crash, wondering if you were dreaming or not. Then the crash comes.

You hear your child's call again, followed closely by sobs.

As you approach her bed, perhaps you hear her coughing, or sniffling hard as she tries to breathe, or moaning as she tells you her tummy hurts. It's a scenario of sickness that for parents is all too common.

"The most common forms of infectious diseases in children are the viral respiratory infections," says Stephen Cochi, M.D., a pediatric epidemiologist at the Centers for Disease Control in Atlanta. "Next come the viruses, bacteria and parasites that cause gastroenteritis and diarrhea."

But when it's *your* child, there is no such thing as a *common* illness—we're talking family here! Experts say there is not much you can do to protect your child from many of the viruses that may be stalking her, but they do say you can fight back.

WINNING THE COLD WAR

Colds, also known as upper respiratory infections, are the biggest enemy when it comes to infecting children. When one strikes your child, and it will, pediatricians say the first counterattack should be fluids. "The first thing the parent must do, what's really important, is to increase the child's intake of fluids," says Paul Baker, M.D., chief of pediatrics at Kaiser-Permanente in Fresno, California.

Long before your child is old enough to hold an orange, good nutrition could be enhancing his immune defenses. Breastfeeding may give the immune system the boost it needs to fight off infections during the first months of life.

"Then attack the symptoms of runny nose, cough and sore throat with over-the-counter decongestants and cough suppressants, given mostly during the night so the child can get rest. Children tend to get over infections more quickly if they're well rested," he says. And you'll be more rested, too.

Dr. Baker says that while there is no known cure for the common cold, and no sure way to prevent it, there is something parents can do to help their children once the cold season arrives.

"Make sure that they are eating well and have a nutritionally balanced diet," he says. "We know for sure that a child with some kind of nutritional deficit—anemia, for example—is more susceptible to these kinds of infections than a child who eats properly."

If your child has a sore throat, though, getting him to eat may be a chore that's hard to swallow. Dr. Baker says that if a school-age child has a sore throat and fever, it's best to see a doctor. "Physicians have a diagnostic kit that lets them identify streptococcal bacteria from the throat. Within 30 minutes of the test, they can tell if it's a strep infection. If it is, penicillin or other antibiotics can be used to treat it."

AN EARFUL OF TROUBLE

If you call your child to come and take his cold medicine, and he ignores you, maybe it's not because the medicine tastes like strawberry. Perhaps he can't hear you clearly because of an ear infection.

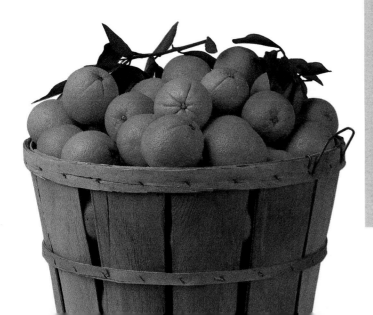

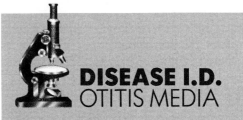

DISEASE I.D.
OTITIS MEDIA

DESCRIPTION: An ear infection, or fluid in the ear, that's usually caused by a virus but can also be from bacteria. It inflames the cells of the middle ear cavity, and it frequently occurs when there is an upper respiratory infection.

INCIDENCE: The number of acute cases in one recent year numbered more than 9.5 million, with 53 percent of children under 5 years old suffering with it.

MODES OF TRANSMISSION: Usually occurs as a secondary infection from an upper respiratory infection. *Hemophilus influenzae* and *Streptococcus pneumoniae* are the most common infectious agents.

DEFENSE FACTORS: Breastfeeding bolsters the child's developing immune system and may help prevent infections of the middle ear. One study found that no breastfed baby developed otitis media before the age of 6 months.

TREATMENT: See your physician. Antibiotics are used for three to six months. If a child still has many ear infections, surgery can be done to insert tubes into the eardrum. The tubes allow air to reach the middle ear and also help to drain the fluid that is clogging the eustachian tube in the ear.

RECOVERY TIME: On antibiotics, the pain and fever should subside in 24 to 48 hours. The fluid may remain for four to six weeks. Surgery should bring almost immediate relief.

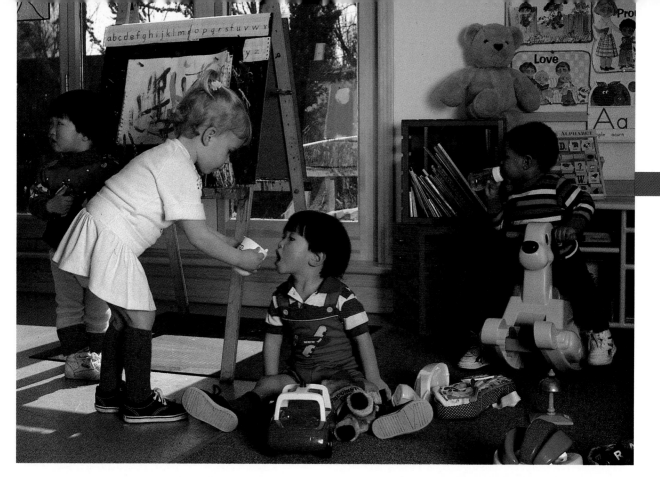

Otitis media, or infection of the middle ear, is a secondary problem associated with upper respiratory infections. "It frequently occurs when a child has a cold," says Kenneth Grundfast, M.D., chairman of the Department of Otolaryngology at the Children's Hospital National Medical Center in Washington, D.C., and coauthor of the book, *Ear Infections in Your Child*.

"In the United States, ear infections are the second most frequent reason for visits to a pediatrician's office. By the age of 2, a typical child will have had approximately three ear infections," Dr. Grundfast says.

Symptoms include fever, crying, restlessness, loss of sleep, tugging at the ear and rubbing the side of the face. There may also be drainage from the ear. Dr. Grundfast says there are things you can do at home to help your child: "Give a nonaspirin pain reliever, apply warm towels to the sore ear and just try to calm and comfort your child. Usually, a visit to the physician is advisable, and an antibiotic may be prescribed."

Pay close attention to that nonaspirin pain relief advice. Pediatric experts agree that because of the aspirin-associated risk of Reye's syndrome (see the box "Every Parent's Nightmare") in children, it's best to substitute acetaminophen when trying to relieve their pain and fever.

Toys aren't the only things that children pass to each other. They also pass along infections. Experts say children in day care seem to get more infections than children who stay at home. Look for a center that's clean, and one where the employees wash their hands after changing a diaper or wiping a nose.

A FEVER PITCH

When things heat up around the house, the experts say, you should bring out the nonaspirin fire brigade quickly. When it comes to treating your child's fever, the response tends to vary by degrees. "A temperature of 104°F isn't going to hurt a 4-, 5- or 6-year-old, but usually they feel miserable enough that you should give them acetaminophen," says Birt Harvey, M.D., professor of pediatrics, Stanford University School of Medicine. "If the temperature is low grade, around 101° or 102°F, unless they feel awful, you don't really need to treat it," he adds.

One way to tell if the child needs treatment is to watch him instead of the thermometer. "Let the child seek his own level of activity," says Edgar Marcuse, M.D., director of ambulatory care at Children's Hospital and Medical Center in Seattle and member of the Committee on Infectious Diseases of the American Academy of Pediatrics.

"Dress him lightly and provide plenty of fluids.

EVERY PARENT'S NIGHTMARE

Parents don't have nightmares about monsters in the closet or the bogeyman under the bed. They wake up sweating after dream encounters with real-life menaces, like meningitis, encephalitis or pneumonia.

Compared with them, a runny nose looks good. Stephen Cochi, M.D., says that these are among the illnesses that can threaten the life of your child and that require immediate medical attention.

Here's his cast of characters for the monsters lurking in parents' dreams.

Encephalitis. An uncommon but very serious infection of the brain tissue, encephalitis is usually caused by a virus. Children develop a high fever and show marked alteration in their mental status. They can become semicomatose, lose their orientation or become very combative. There's often very little to do for it but offer supportive treatment in the hospital, although some forms may respond to drug therapy.

Epiglottiditis. An uncommon bacterial infection, this tends to occur in children 2 to 4 years old. The bacteria enter the bloodstream and infect the soft tissue that covers the windpipe. The tissue swells and starts to cut off the air supply. The child has difficulty breathing, sounds hoarse, may drool excessively and may have a barking, crouplike cough. Hospitalization and antibiotics are required. Sometimes a plastic tube is inserted into the windpipe to aid breathing.

Meningitis. This is an infection of the covering of the brain and the spinal fluid. It's relatively uncommon, with about 20,000 cases reported a year. Bacterial meningitis is the life-threatening kind. The symptoms are very high fever, stiffness of the neck and irritability. In a young infant, the soft spot on the head can bulge. Meningitis needs to be treated in a hospital with antibiotics. There is likely to be a vaccine soon for young infants to prevent some forms of meningitis; there is one now for children older than a year and a half.

Pertussis. Although rare, some 2,500 cases a year of pertussis, also known as whooping cough, are still reported, despite routine use of the DPT vaccination. It is a cough that continues on and on without interruption—long enough that children have a hard time catching their breath. Their faces get blue. They may even vomit or choke. Treatment for pertussis is antibiotics and hospitalization.

Pneumonia. This is an infection of the lung tissue caused by a variety of different organisms, bacterial or viral. The child increases his breathing rate and has difficulty breathing. There is also fever and a cough that may or may not be productive. Treatment is usually with antibiotics.

Reye's syndrome. This is basically a form of encephalitis. Aspirin can be a facilitator of this complication, which is generally associated with influenza virus or chicken pox. Aspirin doesn't cause it but helps it along if either of these two viruses are present. Symptoms include drowsiness, vomiting, personality change and disorientation or confusion. You can help prevent it by giving aspirin substitutes to children under 18 years of age for pain and fever.

Sepsis. It's a blood-borne infection, usually bacterial, that spreads throughout the body. The child has a high fever, chills, fatigue and lack of appetite, and may even go into shock. Hospitalization and antibiotics are the only treatment.

Dr. Cochi stresses that these infectious diseases need expert care. If you suspect your child is suffering with any of them, seek medical attention right away.

His activity will show you how sick he is," says Dr. Marcuse. "But if the fever persists for more than a day or so with no apparent explanation, then you should see your doctor. If your child is under 6 months old and has a fever, you should see your doctor promptly."

INTESTINAL TURMOIL

Just when you think you've taken care of all the things that can go wrong in the upper part of your child's body, the lower part wants its turn. Gastroenteritis and diarrhea are common problems for most youngsters.

Now before you wash your hands of any responsibility, consider this. It seems that to a certain extent these infectious diseases can be prevented through hand washing. "Many times children will be infected by persons who transmit the disease to them because they didn't wash their hands after taking care of another child," says Richard Katz, M.D., a pediatric gastroenterologist at San Diego's Children's Hospital.

This carelessness usually happens at day care centers. "The *Giardia* parasite is endemic to day care centers," says Dr. Katz. "*Giardia* is a very common cause of chronic diarrhea in children, and careful hygiene is one way to prevent its spread."

A physician needs to test the child for this form of diarrhea, and if the test is positive, *Giardia* can be treated with antibiotics. For other types of diarrhea, Dr. Katz recommends giving plenty of fluids so the child won't become dehydrated during the course of the acute attack, which normally lasts three or four days.

THE ITCH OF CHICKEN POX

Parenthood is not for the chicken-hearted, especially since childhood is the time for chicken pox. "It begins with a fever and little lesions or spots that look like dewdrops on a rose petal," says Dr. Marcuse.

To Stanford's Dr. Harvey, the rash initially looks like mosquito bites. He adds, "The rash starts on the face and trunk and then spreads out to the extremities. In two or three days the initial lesions develop a crust, so you see lesions in different stages on the body. The child is considered contagious as long as there are fluid-filled blisters, which is usually five or six days."

About all you can do to treat the disease is to help control the itching. Dr. Harvey recommends a topical anti-itch product like calamine lotion. "In addition, giving the child a bath in a tepid tub with baking soda or cornstarch added may decrease the itching."

Although there is no cure for the disease, a vaccine to prevent chicken pox is being tested. Vaccines for many other childhood illnesses have been around for years. According to the experts, they are effective in more than 90 percent of children. If you're wondering when your child needs vaccinations, refer to the box "When to Immunize."

MEASLES AND MUMPS

Sometimes though, a child will catch a disease even after being immunized. Rare as it is, your child still could catch measles or mumps, for example.

Measles and mumps are both viral infections. Measles begins much like a cold, and needs to be diagnosed by a doctor. But Dr. Marcuse says that if the disease is being reported in the community, parents can look out for some signs. "The child will have a runny nose, cough and red eyes, followed three days later by high fever and a generalized rash that usually begins on the face and neck. The entire illness lasts about ten days."

Mumps is easier to distinguish. Dr. Baker says to look by your child's ear. "The swelling is usually right in front of the ear, first on one side and then the other. The parotid gland swells and actually makes the bottom of the ears protrude from the head."

There is not much you can do once your child has either of these diseases except make him comfortable till the illness runs its course.

WHEN TO IMMUNIZE

Vaccinations have all but eliminated what were once common childhood diseases. Stephen Cochi, M.D., says most childhood vaccinations are 95 to 98 percent effective. "During the peak polio epidemic years of 1951 through 1955, 10,000 to 21,000 cases were reported per year. With the advent of the polio vaccine, only five to ten cases have been reported in recent years," he says. Many younger pediatricians report never having seen mumps, rubella, diphtheria, tetanus, pertussis or polio.

Here's a list of vaccinations, along with the schedule for when the child should receive them. Most are mandatory for all children enrolled in U.S. public schools.

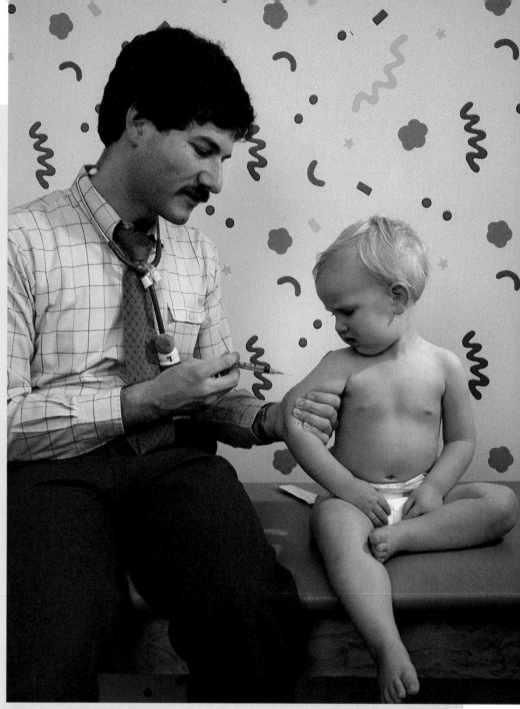

MANDATORY (required by law)

	1ST	BOOSTERS
DPT (diphtheria, pertussis, tetanus)	2, 4, 6 months	18 months, 4 to 6 years
Poliomyelitis	2, 4 months	18 months, 4 to 6 years
TB (tuberculosis) test	1 year	
Measles	15 months	
Mumps	15 months	
Rubella	15 months	
Tetanus-diphtheria		14 to 16 years and every 10 years thereafter

OPTIONAL (but recommended)

	1ST
(HIB) Hemophilus	18 months

COMING SOON

Chicken pox (varicella) vaccine—Still being tested.

Pertussis (whooping cough) vaccine—It is hoped that a new vaccine under development will have fewer side effects than the current DPT vaccine.

DETECTING INFECTION

Kenneth hoists his pale, tired body up on the paper-covered examining table. His complaint? Swollen glands, low-grade fever, fatigue—the very symptoms, in fact, that have been bothering the patient in the next examining room and countless other people in the community.

The diagnosis? Not long ago, the doctor's initial response might have been, "You've got the flu" or "You've got a viral infection." And Kenneth would have been sent home with a prescription for penicillin or another standard antibiotic.

Nowadays, however, many doctors are taking a more sophisticated approach to sleuthing infections. They realize that many infectious illnesses that look alike may be caused by very different culprits. And that means that they can't always be nabbed by the old standby treatments.

Take, for example, the case of mononucleosis, a disease caused by the Epstein-Barr virus. "Mono is a dead ringer for strep throat," says Richard Belsey, M.D., professor of clinical pathology at the Oregon Health Sciences Center in Portland. "In a routine exam, it looks just like strep—people have a sore throat, swollen glands, fever, fatigue."

But there's an important difference. Antibiotics can knock out the streptococci bacteria that can cause strep throat. If it's a virus like mono, on the other hand, such drugs are useless.

To pin down suspicious infections, doctors have traditionally sent specimens of blood, urine, mucus or other tissue to labs. There, technicians put the infected cells in a "culture"—test tubes or petri dishes containing special "food"—and stake out the site to see which infectious organisms grow.

Unfortunately, by the time results are reported back to the doctor, the infection has had plenty of time to do its dirty work.

SPEEDIER DETECTION

Now, faster checks called antigen detection tests are helping doctors become supersleuths at nailing infection. Using cell samples, they can detect the presence of specific antigens (infectious agents) inside the body. The diagnosis is available within minutes.

These rapid tests help doctors blow the cover on a whole range of infections. They can also spot such things as herpes as well as a lesser known sexually transmitted disease called chlamydia. They scope out the bacterial, viral and fungal diseases—even infections like Lyme disease, caused by protozoa.

"The antigen tests are helping doctors become better Sherlock Holmeses," Dr. Belsey says. "We continue to pick up our best clues from the patient interview and the clinical exam. But the new antigen detection tests are like an eyewitness coming in with new evidence."

That evidence can also help you get proper treatment to arrest the disease. "We've got a whole new breed of antiviral drugs that are specific for each disease," explains Jeffrey Galpin, M.D., associate professor of clinical medicine at UCLA and director of the Porton Medical Lab and Clinic.

The herpes virus, for example, can be controlled with acyclovir (Zovirax). Yet this same drug won't do a thing to bacteria, such as mycoplasma, which requires tetracycline. "The antigen tests help you get a correct match," says Dr. Galpin.

But perhaps the most dramatic plus for these rapid antigen detection tests is this: They can actually spot an infection before there are any outward signs of disease.

That means they can pinpoint the Typhoid Marys in the crowd—"the carriers of diseases who show no symptoms," says Albert Balows, Ph.D., assistant director of lab sciences at the Centers for Disease Control in Atlanta.

Chlamydia, for example, is a sexually transmitted infection that affects up to five million women each year and can lead to infertility. But up to 40 percent of these women have silent symptoms—they don't know they have the disease or that they can pass it on. "The antigen test for chlamydia, which a doctor now can perform in the office, makes it possible to detect the disease in a few hours," says Dr. Balows. "That could spare countless others from infection."

NEW AGE OF THERMOMETERS

Move over mercury. Modern science has finally come up with something to beat the centuries-old fever detector, the mercury-in-glass thermometer.

"It's still the gold standard in temperature taking," says Leonard Banco, M.D., associate professor of pediatrics, University of Connecticut School of Medicine. But many people haven't learned to use it properly. They have trouble reading the sliver of mercury against those tiny tick lines. They wonder how long to keep the thermometer in, what happens if it slips in the mouth, or worse, if it breaks.

For the record, the proper way to take an adult's temperature is to first shake the thermometer so the mercury is below 96°F. Then place the thermometer under the tongue for 2 to 3 minutes. A fever may range from 100° to 104°F for a few days, depending on the time of day, the activity level, whether hot or cold foods have just been eaten, and where the thermometer is placed in the mouth. Shivering means the fever is peaking, sweating means it's coming down. And no, you won't get mercury poisoning if the glass breaks.

You may want to consider these "new-fangled" thermometers to make the job easier:

Digital thermometers. These plastic, paddle-shaped devices have a sensor in the tip that sends electrical signals to the thermometer's tiny computer chip. In about a minute, a beep alerts you to a number displayed in the window. Digitals are quick and easy to read, and there's no need to shake them. The drawback? The battery may give out just when you need it most.

Electronic thermometers. Popular in hospitals and doctors' offices, these high-tech thermometers are now available for home use. They consist of a steel probe that resembles the glass thermom-

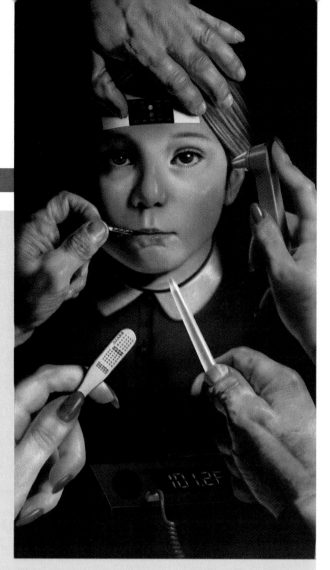

eter except that inside is a supersensing device called a thermistor. The probe is attached with a cord to a monitor and when the probe is placed under the tongue, the monitor flashes a digital readout in mere seconds. Plus, the probes are covered with disposable plastic sheaths so there's no risk of infection.

Forehead strips. Remember the mood ring? Same idea. Reusable plastic strips impregnated with liquid crystals are affixed to the forehead and change colors with temperature changes. They're lots of fun, but not so accurate. Why? Foreheads are not very good indicators of core body temperature. The strips may also be thrown off by cold hands or cool rooms.

Urinary thermometers. This device may be useful for charting ovulation. A urine sample is collected in a disposable cup outfitted with a temperature-sensing device. Supposedly, the advantage is that urine temperatures don't vary as much as oral temperatures.

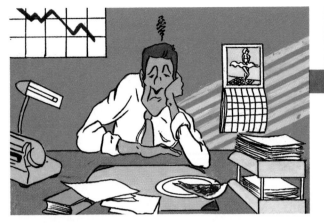

You're so wiped out, it's an effort to tell the doc what hurts. You feel like you've been broadsided by a truck. Your cheeks are flushed and your throat is so raw that eating pizza is like swallowing glass. Your mind is muddled, your co-workers act like you've got the plague and you can't afford any downtime. Help!

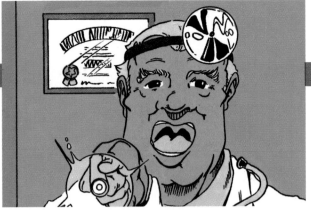

Say a-ahh . . . The doctor shines his beam onto a crimson throat dotted with ugly white patches. He feels walnut-size lymph nodes and watches the mercury shoot up on the thermometer. His suspicion? Strep throat. If he's right, you'll need an antibiotic before it turns into something nastier, like rheumatic fever.

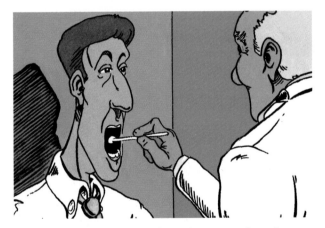

Luckily, your doctor can take a throat swab to detect strep while you wait. No need to wait for a specimen to finish "cooking" in a culture in some lab. The swab is simply placed in a solution containing latex beads coated with antibodies. If the strep bacteria are present, they'll "clump" with the antibodies.

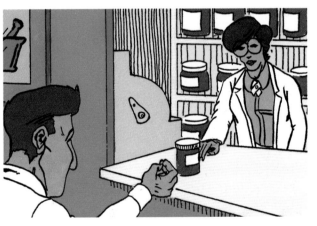

Ten minutes later: Your strep test is positive. And the good news? You can take an antibiotic today and be able to eat pizza tomorrow. You'll no longer be feared as a carrier of germs. Best of all, this rapid strep test—and rapid treatment—saves your immune system from working overtime to battle the infection.

HOW TO "READ" A VIRUS

Different antigen tests detect different infections. One type, the fluorescent antibody (FA) test, uses special dyes to expose diseases like respiratory infections. Nasal secretions are sent to a lab, where they are affixed to a slide and stained with dye. The slide is placed under a microscope and read to see which viruses show up. Test results are available within a few hours. The drawback? These tests require costly equipment and highly trained personnel.

But newer rapid antigen detection tests are about as simple to do as a pregnancy test.

These tests are based on the fact that if antigens of a disease are present, they will cause infection-fighting antibodies to react by clumping, or agglutinating, with the antigen. Antigen agglutination tests make this clumping visible.

In one such test, antibodies or antigens are

coated with latex beads to expose clumping. The test is commonly used to detect bacterial or fungal infections. And it's fast, detecting strep throat in 15 minutes.

One of the most sensitive agglutination tests—especially useful for detecting the Epstein-Barr virus, herpes and even AIDS—is called the enzyme-linked immunosorbent assay, or ELISA.

It works like this. The doctor uses a plate or tube to which a custom-made antibody has been attached. Next, a tissue specimen is added. If a viral agent is present, it will clump with the antibody. The clumping is detected when a second antiviral antibody is added, causing a color change. Color indicates the test is positive—the disease is present. Results can be obtained in a few hours or less.

One disadvantage is that the ELISA test can detect only one disease at a time. Doctors have to know in advance what they're looking for, because it requires using disease-specific antibodies.

HOW THE TESTS RATE

How do the new rapid tests compare to cultures? For a test to be rated accurate, explains Dr. Galpin, it must rate high in *sensitivity* (be able to show positive results when a disease is present) and have a low rate of false-positives. It must also rate high in *specificity* (showing a negative result when no disease is present) and have a low rate of false-negatives.

A test's ratings may vary for particular diseases. The strep test, for example, shows a respectable false-positive rate of 44 percent but a troublesome false-negative rate of 78 percent. That means there's a good chance that it'll show you don't have strep when you really do.

"Test results depend on several factors," says Dr. Galpin. Cortisone or antibiotics may mask an infection. Specimens may be improperly prepared or tests incorrectly run, and antibodies may be outdated or inappropriate for the disease.

That's why one positive antigen test is rarely enough to make a diagnosis, and why for certain

HIGH-TECH DETECTION

Detecting some diseases is like looking for a needle in a haystack. Take AIDS, for example. Scientists literally have to look at 150,000 cells to find the single one infected by the virus.

Such painstaking, arduous tasks may become a thing of the past. The state of the art in infection detection is taking place in an unimposing machine much like an incubator. What's cooking? Basically, DNA.

First, an infected cell from a human specimen is broken down. The DNA is taken out and heated, cracking its genetic code. It's then multiplied, making "the needle in the haystack" easier to find. Specifically, the ladderlike double helix of DNA is "unzipped." It's reproduced and a probe containing a genetic code is introduced. When the probe finds its mate, it zips up the DNA and signals that an infection is found.

The plus for the nucleic probe? It's safer than growing dangerous organisms in test tubes. It's also faster, reaping results in a matter of hours. Best of all, the method could be used in a doctor's office, making it easier to stop deadly diseases in their tracks.

tests, doctors recommend that negative tests be checked against a culture to confirm results.

"As super as these rapid antigen tests are," reminds Dr. Belsey, "they are only one part of the diagnosis. Eighty percent of the diagnosis still comes from a careful review of the patient's symptoms and history."

Your test results should be consistent with your symptoms, history and whether you fit into a high-risk group, adds Dr. Belsey. "If a test indicates herpes, for example, and you *know* that you and your spouse have been faithful, have the test repeated and get a culture, too."

DRUGS AND THE IMMUNE SYSTEM

Say no to "bugs": Don't do drugs. The chances of catching the latest infectious bug going around are already high enough for most of us without factoring in the ill effects of illegal drugs. Marijuana, cocaine and other drugs, scientists are discovering, undermine the body's natural resistance to disease.

GETTING LOW FROM A HIGH

Dope smokers may feel high, but their overall health level is pretty low. They get sick more often than nonsmokers, and their respiratory systems are more vulnerable to everything from chronic bronchitis to lung cancer.

"It has been suspected for some time that smoking marijuana harms the immune system," says Eliezer Huberman, Ph.D., senior scientist at the Department of Energy's Argonne National Laboratory. "Only recently have we been able to pinpoint cell types that may be involved."

The maturation of infection-fighting monocytes, for instance, is impeded by marijuana, Dr. Huberman discovered. When a call to arms is issued against invading microbes, fewer mature monocytes are ready to report for duty.

And those monocytes have a rough time of it,

says David Ou, Ph.D., clinical assistant professor of pathology at the University of Illinois and chief of immunology at the Veterans Administration West Side Medical Center in Chicago. Marijuana's primary chemical agent, tetrahydrocannabinol (THC), slows the monocytes down as they march to the battleground, and when they finally get there, they don't have their customary ravenous appetites for the bad guys.

While most studies have been conducted in a test tube, Dr. Ou believes their results accurately apply to real-life marijuana users—who would, by the way, probably benefit immediately if they quit the habit.

CONCERNS ABOUT COCAINE

Used regularly by more than five million Americans, coke hurts the body in numerous ways—some of them deadly—including nasal discomfort and damage, upper respiratory infections, hepatitis, seizures, heart

Are Americans going to pot? Maybe, if they're puffing the cell-damaging stuff shown here—just a tiny patch of the $10 billion a year marijuana industry that outgrosses lettuce or tomatoes.

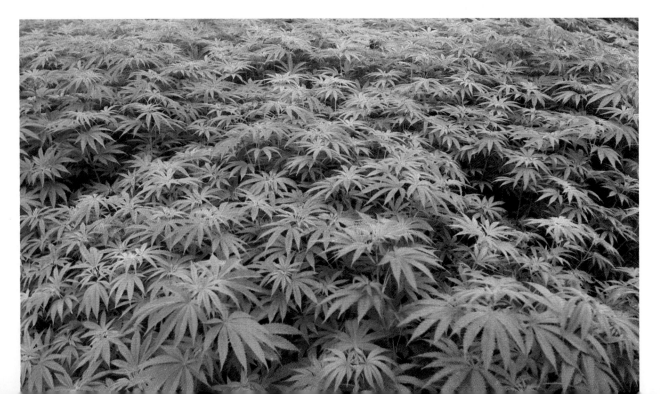

attacks and strokes. Crack, a form of coke that is smoked rather than sniffed, is no less hazardous.

Research on cocaine's interactions with immunity is relatively recent and far from conclusive. A study by a team of scientists at Temple University School of Medicine suggested that low levels of cocaine did not suppress but actually enhanced the immune response of laboratory mice. The researchers theorize, however, that because cocaine's effects take hold and then recede rather quickly, the results might have been different had they given the mice the drug on a more continuous basis—the same way many coke users take it.

The amount of cocaine taken apparently makes a difference. Studying laboratory animals injected with the drug, "we found that phagocytosis—or the ability of phagocyte cells to engulf invading microbes —decreases substantially," Dr. Ou says. "But the size of this decrease depends on how much cocaine is injected and when."

What's more, Dr. Ou's study established a cumulative effect: Whether an animal was given a large amount of cocaine on one day or one-fourth that amount over a period of four days, the animal's phagocytes were equally depleted.

Dr. Ou also found that after ten days, tumors in animals given cocaine seemed to grow larger than tumors in cocaine-free animals, suggesting that the drug interferes with the body's natural defenses against cancer.

DEADLY STREET DRUGS

Amphetamines (diet pills or "speed"), heroin and the vast variety of synthetic street drugs can expose their users to everything from murderously high fevers to Parkinson's disease, a form of muscular paralysis. Drug use may even interact with the AIDS virus. Butyl nitrite sniffing by homosexuals, theorize some scientists, may induce Kaposi's sarcoma, a deadly tumor once common among AIDS victims.

If there's one habit that's always worth breaking, it's drugs. If you do them, drop them—before they break you.

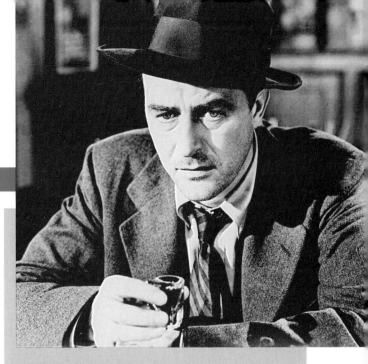

THE HARD FACTS ABOUT HARD DRINKING

Down-and-out Don Birnam, portrayed by actor Ray Milland in the classic film *The Lost Weekend*, is a loser on more than one count. Not only is he an alcoholic—one of an estimated ten million in this country—but his habit puts his health at tremendous risk.

Excessive use of alcohol, either in binges or on a more regular basis, has been linked to heart disease; high blood pressure; digestive disturbances; cirrhosis of the liver; cancer of the mouth, esophagus and breast; brain damage; malnutrition and sexual impotence, among other problems.

How is it that people who seem to spend so much time drinking to one another's health turn out to be so sickly? The poisons they're pouring damage their overall immunity to disease, medical researchers believe.

Alcoholics have low levels of granulocytes, for instance. These immune system cells have the task of hightailing it to infected areas of the body to eat up invading microbes before they get a chance to spread to the rest of the body. As a result, organs like the lungs and the liver perform their protective job more slowly when there is alcohol on the scene. Also, alcohol ingestion interferes with the body's production of antibodies against any new infections.

In other words, drinking and thriving just don't mix.

EMERGENCY INFECTIONS

What's the first thing that comes to mind when you think of hospital emergency rooms? A head-on collision? A tumble out of a tree? A knife that slipped?

The business of emergency medical care isn't always so bloody. In fact, sometimes there's no blood at all. From 15 to 30 percent of all admissions involve infections, not trauma, according to Michael Tomlanovich, M.D., head of the Department of Emergency Medicine at Detroit's Henry Ford Hospital.

WHEN THE BODY SCREAMS "UNCLE!"

You already know what an emergency is: a situation demanding immediate action—or else. And you know what an infection is: an invasion of the body. So what exactly is an emergency infection? Sorry, you won't find it in *Webster's Dictionary*. According to Emily Lucid, M.D., director of the Division of Emergency Medicine at Pittsburgh's Allegheny Hospital, "Emergency is in the eye of the beholder. You've got to define it in your own terms."

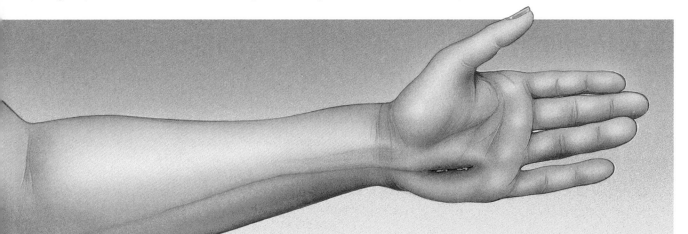

SURE SIGN OF INFECTION

Often it is called blood poisoning. But red streaks, like the one you see in this illustration, are no more blood poisoning than a jellyfish is a fish or a pineapple an apple. Yet that's what it's often called.

True, those red streaks emanating from a localized infection (usually a cut) do indicate the infection is spreading. And yes, you'd better get help right away. But the infection is *not* spreading through your blood. It's moving through the intricate network of tiny vessels that make up your lymphatic system.

The condition is lymphangitis. You may have heard the old yarn about the streaks traveling to your heart and when they get there, you die. "It's not like that," says Earl Schwartz, M.D. The infection has no interest in racing to your ticker. Rather, it's moving toward the closest lymph nodes. (On your arm, as shown above, that would be inside your elbow and armpit.)

As serious as lymphangitis is, *real* blood poisoning is much more dangerous. In the old days, a victim of the condition that doctors call septicemia often died within hours. Today, thanks to antibiotics, it's no longer invariably fatal. Symptoms of septicemia are a rapid rise in temperature, chills, fatigue and paleness. The disease can result from any untreated infection, including lymphangitis, but more commonly from urinary tract infections or pneumonia, says Dr. Schwartz.

That is, what constitutes a medical emergency for one person may not seem like—may not *be*—an emergency for another. "Diseases that may not be serious in a healthy individual may become serious in a person who is immunologically compromised," says Dr. Lucid. Such compromised individuals, she says, include those with lymphoma (a tumor of the lymphatic system), leukemia or diabetes, those whose spleens have been removed, the very elderly, AIDS patients and—when it comes to respiratory infections—smokers. For these folks, a case of common flu or even a common cold can sometimes spell big trouble. Be advised, if you're in one of these groups, to treat all infections with respect.

How about those of us who are otherwise bursting with health? "Most infections that are going to cause trouble linger before reaching a critical stage. You seldom get a life-threatening infection that hits you all at once," says Earl Schwartz, M.D., associate professor of emergency medicine at the Bowman Gray School of Medicine at Wake Forest University in Winston-Salem, North Carolina.

The few infections that really can be lethal almost from the word "go" are rare, says Dr. Schwartz. They include rabies, tetanus, peritonitis and the central nervous system infections—encephalitis and meningitis. The next closest thing to true emergency infections are those which, left untreated, may become life-threatening in time. These include pneumonia, urinary tract infections, certain skin infections, tonsillitis and infections of the ears, nose and eyes.

SIGNS OF TROUBLE BREWING

Many of the infections people consider emergencies really aren't, says Dr. Tomlanovich. On the other hand, some infections absolutely are emergencies. But how can you tell the true crises from the false alarms?

"We see people all the time who come to the emergency room in bad shape, having missed some

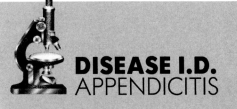

DISEASE I.D.
APPENDICITIS

DESCRIPTION: You should suspect appendicitis if you're experiencing nausea, acute abdominal pain (typically in the lower right part of your gut) and fever. These symptoms often mean your appendix is inflamed and probably infected. Ironically, this little horn-shaped pouch jutting out from the base of your large intestine seems to have no other purpose than to sometimes make your life miserable.

INCIDENCE: In any given year, about 1 person in 500 will suffer an attack of appendicitis.

MODE OF TRANSMISSION: Why the appendix sometimes becomes irritated, swollen and susceptible to infection is not fully understood. It is believed that sometimes an obstruction, such as intestinal worms or a piece of fecal matter, can clog up the organ. The disease is not contagious.

DEFENSE FACTOR: Some researchers believe that a diet high in refined, fiber-deficient foods contributes to the likelihood that you'll get appendicitis. Since inflamed appendixes are often found blocked by hard fecal matter, keeping your stools soft with a high-fiber diet may be a good defense.

TREATMENT: If you suspect appendicitis, see a doctor immediately. *Do not* use laxatives. Once appendicitis is diagnosed, surgery to remove the inflamed appendix is usually required. If not removed, it can rupture, leading to potentially fatal peritonitis (see "Disease I.D.: Peritonitis" on page 25).

RECOVERY TIME: In the hands of a competent surgeon, an appendectomy is a relatively safe and simple operation. You should be back on your feet in a few days.

THE MYSTERY THAT WAS TOXIC SHOCK

In 1980, a rash of deaths from infections related to tampon use sent shock waves throughout America. Toxic shock syndrome soon became a household word.

At first, though, medical researchers were baffled. It wasn't until over 100 cases of the syndrome had been reported that the connection was first made to tampons. More than 150 cases after that, the connection was made to a particular kind of tampon—the newly introduced, highly absorbent, leave-it-in-for-many-hours kind.

In retrospect, it makes sense, says Emily Lucid, M.D. These women died of a bacterial infection—and blood, says Dr. Lucid "is the best culture medium there is for bacteria."

The suspect tampons were removed from the market in September of 1980. But toxic shock syndrome has not been eliminated. The Centers for Disease Control (CDC) estimates an incidence of two to four cases per 100,000 women each year. If you use tampons, your risk of infection will be minimized by choosing the least absorbent one necessary to catch your flow, says Claire Broome, M.D., a researcher with the CDC.

"No matter what type of tampon you use," says Dr. Lucid, "change it regularly. A good way to do that is to change the tampon every time you urinate." And by all means, she says, if you develop a high fever, vomiting, diarrhea and a rash—whether you are menstruating or not—get help fast.

obvious signs of serious infection," says Dr. Schwartz. What are those obvious signs? Here are some symptoms that may spell trouble.

Fever. "Fever is not an illness in itself; it's usually part of your defense against illness. But in general, the more virulent the illness, the more elevated your temperature," says Dr. Tomlanovich. When should you seek medical care? A good rule of thumb to use with fever, as with other general signs of infection (like fatigue, weakness and decreased appetite) is to "ask yourself if the symptoms are debilitating," he says. A debilitating fever, for example, would probably *not* be the 99.5° or 100°F that usually accompanies simple flu, but rather (depending on the individual) a temperature of between 102° and 105°F. "For anything over 105°F you should certainly seek help," he advises.

Cough. If a cold strikes, it's natural to clear your throat with a little hack from time to time. But when your coughing yields phlegm that's cloudy, yellowish, brownish or tinged with blood, or when it's accompanied by chest pain, shortness of breath or fever, then you may have pneumonia. This infection (usually bacterial, though sometimes viral) "has probably killed more people than any other," says Dr. Schwartz. Today, however, rapid treatment with antibiotics will usually set things right.

Sore throat. "If it's a pain like you can't believe," and you've also got fever and swollen glands, see a doctor. You may have tonsillitis, an infection that hits adults as well as kids. Years ago, doctors removed tonsils at the drop of a scalpel. Today these masses of lymphoid tissue are removed only if they give you recurrent trouble. In any case, says Dr. Tomlanovich, a tonsillectomy would never be performed in response to an emergency. Rather, expect relief from antibiotics and topical anesthetics.

Pain or burning during urination. This may be a sign of a urinary tract infection that could lead to bigger trouble, says Dr. Tomlanovich. Other symptoms may include fever and pain in the kidney area. Urinary tract infections are fairly common and are usually readily treatable with antibiotics.

Skin punctures. "You don't need to see a doctor for every little scrape," says Dr. Schwartz. But should you experience redness, swelling or severe pain near a wound, seek help promptly, he says. "We see people who come in with gangrenous tissue that was obviously infected for a long time. They may wind up losing a finger or toe because they waited too long, thinking the infection would go away by itself." Be especially concerned with bites—human as well as animal. Remember that a bite can be inflicted passively. Major infections often result from fistfights, says Dr. Schwartz, in which the punch-happy antagonist walks away with teeth marks—and a colony of dangerous bacteria—in his knuckles.

Earaches. "Ear infections can spread to the brain and spinal cord," says Dr. Schwartz. So any ear pain, whether it's accompanied by fever and discharge of pus or not, should be checked out promptly. Ear infections are usually treatable with antibiotics taken either by mouth or in drops.

Clogged nose. If stuffiness is accompanied by severe headaches and fever, you've likely got a sinus infection, says Dr. Schwartz. Like ear infections, sinus infections can spread. So don't treat them lightly. Antibiotics can clear them up.

Conjunctivitis (pinkeye). This redness, itchiness and crustiness of the eye is very common, and most often, not very serious. At least the viral version isn't serious. There is, however, a bacterial kind that can lead to severe eye damage. It's best to have pinkeye checked out by a physician.

Now that you know what you're looking for, you should be able to spot most infections that require prompt medical care. Distinguishing the emergency infection from the run-of-the-mill variety is largely a matter of listening attentively to subtle signals. "Your body is an amazing organism," says Dr. Tomlanovich. "Pay attention to it, and it'll tell you when it needs help."

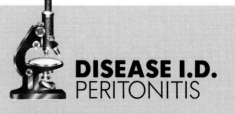

DISEASE I.D.
PERITONITIS

DESCRIPTION: An inflammation of the peritoneum, a double layer of membrane that lines the abdominal cavity and covers the stomach and intestines, peritonitis almost always occurs as a complication of another disease, such as appendicitis, perforated ulcer or alcoholic cirrhosis. Usually, there's severe abdominal pain (which worsens when you move), and the abdomen may feel tender and rigid. Fever, nausea and vomiting may also occur.

INCIDENCE: The disease is rare in countries with adequate medical care. But if treatment for abdominal problems such as appendicitis is delayed, peritonitis is almost inevitable.

MODES OF TRANSMISSION: Peritonitis is caused by infection or irritation from a burst appendix, perforated ulcer or bladder, or ruptured gallbladder or spleen. It is not contagious.

DEFENSE FACTOR: Because this disease is a complication of other disorders, the best defense is to seek medical care at the first sign of any serious stomach or abdominal trouble.

TREATMENT: If peritonitis is neglected, the risks are great, and include death. If you have severe abdominal pain that lasts more than 10 to 20 minutes and is accompanied by any of the symptoms mentioned above, get medical help immediately. Prompt surgery is generally required. Antibiotic therapy is a usual part of treatment.

RECOVERY TIME: Prospects for full recovery from peritonitis are excellent. Recovery time will depend on the nature of the surgery, which may involve removing the appendix or another organ.

FITNESS AND SPORTS

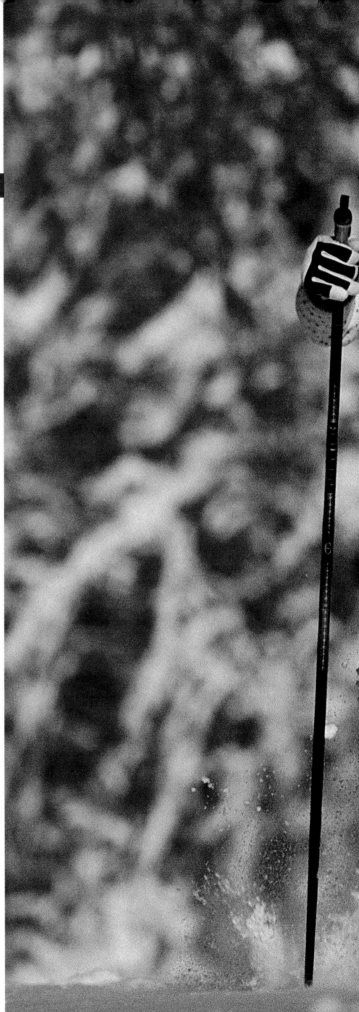

Portrait of a skier in the West:

In the bone-dry air at 10,000 feet, crystals of snow glitter like cut diamonds in the hard light—enormous sparkling strands draped over the pines and blanketing the mountains. There's no wind, but when you're arcing down the side of a mountain at 60 miles an hour, it doesn't matter—you make your own.

You exhale hard at the start of each turn, take a breath during the float while your skis swivel between turns, then let it out again when the edges bite.

A sparkling sheet of snow explodes into the air.

Portrait of a swimmer in the Caribbean:

The sun's hot in a blue sky, and a white-sand beach glitters in the distance. A brisk wind clips the waves, throwing a fine white plume of saltwater into your face each time you roll your head up for air.

You continue to roll and reach with your arms in the stroke called a crawl, and the beach draws closer.

A skier in the Rockies, a swimmer in the Caribbean. Nothing in common, right? Wrong. The people in these portraits have one characteristic they share with one another—and with other men and women who work to stay in shape: An immune system that probably works better than their chair-borne brethren's.

"The impact exercise has on the immune system is not one of those questions where you can point to a set of studies and say, 'this is absolutely proven, beyond question,'" says Robert Jones, Ph.D., director of the Prevention and Health Promotion Program of the Department of Family Medicine at Pennsylvania State University's College of Medicine.

"The evidence simply isn't conclusive. But I'd have to say that, based on research and clinical experience, it's clear that *something* happens to the

Cross-country skiing wins for best all-around aerobic exercise. Research indicates vigorous exercise may also bolster your body's ability to fight off infection.

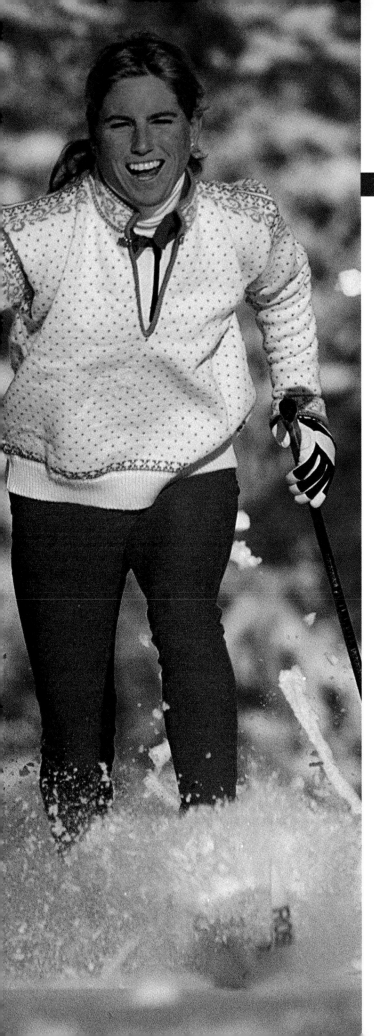

immune system in people who exercise. And I'd have to say that, within certain limits, the effects appear to be positive."

THE EXERCISE EFFECT

The truth is, research exploring the relationship between exercise and immune function—in plain words, your resistance to infection—hasn't reached any clear conclusions.

"With the recent focus on the health benefits of exercise," writes researcher Laurel Traeger Mackinnon, Ph.D., in the *Annals of Sports Medicine*, "it is surprising that relatively little is known about how exercise affects the immune system—despite an interest dating to the early part of this century."

But nonetheless, scientific searchlights have stripped the shadow away from some parts of the puzzle. Current and past research has documented the following effects of moderate exercise on the body's battle system:

• A transient, short-term increase in the number of white blood cells circulating in the bloodstream.

• An increase in antibody and natural killer cell activity.

• Changes in the distribution of circulating lymphocytes—a special subgroup of white blood cells—within the body.

• Increases in plasma levels of interleukin-1, a substance that amplifies the production of immune cells.

What does it all mean? Well, don't panic if you're not sure. At this point, even the professionals are uncertain. "The problem we have in evaluating this information is that the studies aren't clear on what these changes mean for the effectiveness of the immune system," Dr. Jones says. "But some studies are absolutely better than others, and just because you've got six that say one thing and only one that says something else, that doesn't mean that one study is wrong—it all depends on how well they're put together. You have to pick and choose carefully," he says.

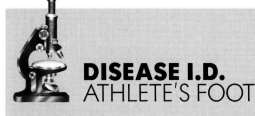

DISEASE I.D.
ATHLETE'S FOOT

DESCRIPTION: A fungal infection of the feet, typically occurring in the webbed tissue between the fourth and fifth toes on each foot. Produces redness, inflammation, scaling and itching.

INCIDENCE: Common in locker rooms, health clubs and other athletic facilities—in general, wherever people exercise and take showers afterward.

MODE OF TRANSMISSION: Direct contact is required. Active men and women typically get athlete's foot by stepping on fungal spores in the locker room or shower area.

DEFENSE FACTORS: Wearing shower shoes is probably the best defense, closely followed by keeping your feet dry. Try using one of the many available foot powders to keep the toe area moisture free. Also, wear socks and shoes that breathe, such as leather.

TREATMENT: Usually, an antifungal cream, like Tinactin or Micatin, applied according to package directions and careful attention to keeping your feet dry. Problem cases can be treated with griseofulvin tablets, which will eliminate those infections that don't respond to topical creams. Meanwhile, an over-the-counter antihistamine can help relieve a mean itch.

RECOVERY TIME: With treatment, recovery will take three to four weeks.

"Threshholds of some sort seem to be involved, which fits with the way the body works generally. On the one end, you've got the sedentary person whose immune system may be depressed from not doing enough. On the other end, you've got the overtrained athlete whose immune system may be down from doing too much.

"I think there's probably a healthful level of exercise somewhere in the middle that does enhance the immune system. Again, exactly how or how much aren't questions we can answer right now with scientific validity. But boosting seems to require moderate to medium exercise sustained over a period of time—years, for example, instead of months."

How do you know whether you're doing enough and not too much? Dr. Jones offers a simple rule of thumb for deciding when to put the pedal to the metal and when to hit the brakes.

"You ought to feel *more* energetic when you're through, not less," he says. "Your mood should be up, buoyed, not down. You should have the feeling that you're enjoying yourself. If you're not, chances are you're working too hard."

HAZARDS IN THE ARENA

Okay, it's good for you—so what else is new?

Well, try this on for size: The virus responsible for herpes—the kind you *don't* want to get—can live for up to 5 hours on the edge of a pool or the rim of a hot tub.

And you thought it was safe to go back in the water.

Exercise may have good effects on your immune system—but what kinds of infection risks are you running when you try to take advantage of that?

Athlete's foot. "Absolutely rampant in health clubs and gyms, this is simply a fungus that causes scaling, itching and redness," says nationally known sports physician Gabe Mirkin, M.D. "You can usually tell when it's athlete's foot by looking at the location: If the tops of your toes are red and inflamed, it's probably just abrasion and pressure from the shoe. If it's dispersed over the bottom of the foot, it's

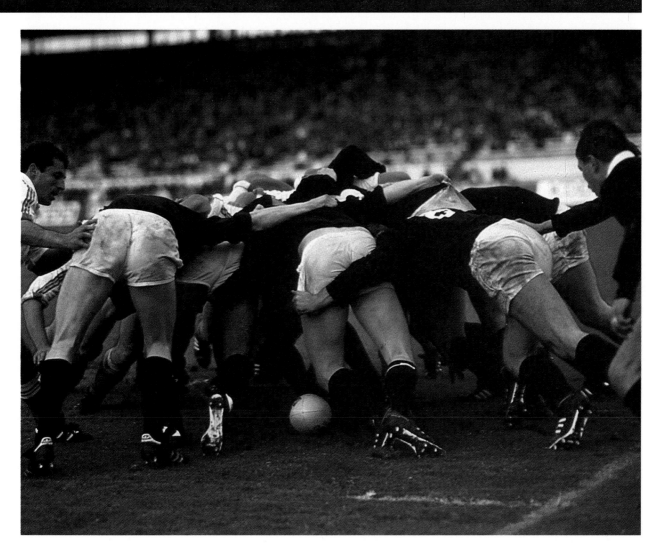

probably a skin disease of some sort.

"But you usually find athlete's foot in the dampest, darkest spots possible, almost always the spaces between the fourth and fifth toes." (For additional information, see the box "Disease I.D.: Athlete's Foot".)

Ringworm. This is another common locker room fungal infection. Like athlete's foot, it is transmitted through contact with the fungus—either on another person or on something they've rubbed against. Ringworm is named for the circular patches of red, scaling skin it produces. Dr. Mirkin says positive diagnosis requires laboratory tests, since

Rugby is a tough, virile sport—but unlike some other tough, virile sports, it can lead to infection with herpes simplex virus. A study by University of Connecticut researchers documented four cases in which rugby players developed herpes infections, apparently from contact with infected teammates.

many other infections mimic ringworm. But treatment is simple—typically, use of a good over-the-counter antifungal cream like Tinactin or Mycelex.

Molluscum contagiosum. This sounds sinister, especially when you find out that it's caused by a virus similar to herpes. But it's actually a relatively

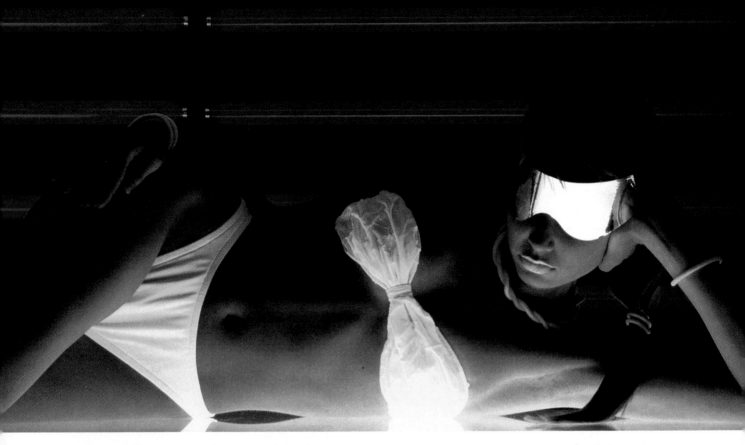

An artificial tan may make you look healthier, but that beautiful bronze glow may be more trouble than it's worth. A number of human and animal studies indicate that ultraviolet radiation can suppress your immune system. Possible results: more frequent infections.

harmless viral infection that generates wartlike bumps in the affected areas. It occurs most often in wrestlers and other contact athletes, in areas of high contact like the underarms and shoulders. Dr. Mirkin says treatment is just a matter of finding a physician to scrape off the bumps.

Herpes gladiatorum. Another infection common among wrestlers and football players, this member of the herpes family produces the blister clusters that characterize the clan. Dr. Mirkin says that, unlike herpes simplex or genital herpes, *Herpes gladiatorum* often may not recur if the initial bout doesn't produce blisters near the mouth or other openings in

the skin. But it's nothing to take lightly, since an attack can last six weeks and produce blister clusters over large areas of the body.

"A very safe treatment is available that often shortens the term of the disease," according to Dr. Mirkin. It's Zovirax (a brand name for acyclovir) taken five times a day for ten days. This often shortens the course of these blisters to just days instead of weeks.

Dr. Mirkin offers the following more general suggestions for minimizing your risks in locker rooms and fitness clubs:

● Don't sit unprotected on toilet seats, locker room benches or sauna platforms. Wear shorts or use a towel to protect against herpes.

● Don't walk barefoot. Use shower shoes to cut the risk of athlete's foot.

● Don't share clothes or towels, which can act as transmitters for skin infections.

● Wear gloves if you lift weights (to prevent warts).

WHEN TO CANCEL EXERCISE

Occasionally, the best way to protect your health is to know when to skip exercise entirely. Whether caused by a virus or generated by proliferating bacteria, a sore throat needs to be cared for—and Dr. Mirkin cautions that every sore throat should be taken seriously.

"If you have a severely sore throat, see a doctor," he says. "The reason you want to treat *all* sore throats is simply because a certain percentage are caused by strep. Strep can cause rheumatic fever and glomerulonephritis—conditions that may damage the heart and kidneys permanently."

His recommendation, especially if a fever accompanies your sore throat: Do *not* exercise.

Instead, see your doctor and get it treated. A common medical treatment for strep throat is penicillin. And one definition of mononucleosis, a viral infection that can mimic strep early on, is simply a sore throat that doesn't respond to penicillin. But mono shares one other characteristic with strep: It is potentially lethal.

"The reason you have to stop exercising if your doctor gives you a diagnosis of mononucleosis is because the spleen and liver enlarge when you have it," Dr. Mirkin says. "A hard blow to your belly could rupture the spleen and kill you."

Beyond rest and recuperation, there's no effective treatment for mononucleosis.

The flu bug, which strikes so many every year, is often treated with fluids and rest, much as mono is. And like mono, it's an indicator against exercise.

"You shouldn't exercise when you've got the flu, with fever and aching muscles," Dr. Mirkin says. "The virus affects the muscles, and if you try to exercise, you're more likely to tear them. And when you have a fever, your heart has to work harder. Since it's a muscle also, the virus can affect it, too. It's highly unlikely, but you could develop an irregular heartbeat and die."

Dr. Mirkin emphasizes that any viral infection can have a similar result if you insist on exercising despite feeling under the weather.

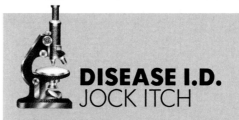

DISEASE I.D.
JOCK ITCH

DESCRIPTION: Comes in three varieties. The first variety is caused by chafing or rubbing and typically results in a bright red, nonscaly (smooth) rash with sharp borders. The second variety is the result of fungal infection and is typically dull red and ring shaped with scaly edges. The scrotum is usually unaffected. The third variety is produced by yeast bacteria, which generate bright red, scaling patches that are irregularly shaped. The patches are accompanied by a bright red, shiny scrotum.

INCIDENCE: Fairly common, with chafing being responsible most often, followed by fungal and then yeast infections.

MODE OF TRANSMISSION: Direct contact with a contaminated surface. Jock itch can also be an allergic reaction to things such as underwear.

DEFENSE FACTORS: Keeping groin area clean and dry. Wearing loose-fitting clothing that doesn't bind in the groin.

TREATMENT: Powder and cortisone creams for chafing. Antifungal creams like Tinactin or Micatin can be used when fungal or yeast infections are involved. Castellani Paint, available only by prescription, works well on yeast infections.

RECOVERY TIME: Varies, from several days to several weeks, depending on the cause and severity of the inflammation.

FOOD

If you ever get to a fancy restaurant in Tokyo and are in the mood for something daring, look for *fugu* on the menu. If you've still got a yen after eyeing the price, and you're feeling bold—real bold— go ahead and order it. But know that one bite from sloppily prepared *fugu* and you can say sayonara to this world.

It takes about ½ milligram—the tiniest speck—of the poison found in the liver and sex organs of the *fugu* (pufferfish) to kill you. For this reason, *fugu* must be prepared by licensed chefs, highly trained in surgically removing the fish's vile toxin. But like real surgeons, they sometimes slip. And some Japanese foolishly try to prepare the fish at home. About 100 *fugu* fans die each year. The final death toll then includes the occasional faulty *fugu* chef, who, shamed by his fatal blunder, commits hara-kiri.

In this country, few people kill themselves over ill-prepared food. But ill-prepared food can, and

occasionally does, kill. Not to worry—food-poisoning deaths in America, as in all developed countries, including Japan, are rare. But problems like diarrhea, cramps and vomiting from "something I ate" are not so rare. The very young, the very old and those with weakened immune systems are more likely to be hit severely—but anyone can be at risk. The Food and Drug Administration (FDA) estimates that as many as one American in six may fall prey to food poisoning each year.

Ill-prepared *fugu*, of course, is poisonous by its very nature. So are the wrong kinds of wild mushrooms. (Poisonous mushrooms take one or two lives in America per year.) Much more often, though, when eating something results in death or illness, it's not really the food itself that's to blame. Instead, the culprits are microorganisms that have temporarily set up housekeeping in that otherwise innocuous slice of chicken, ham or coconut custard pie.

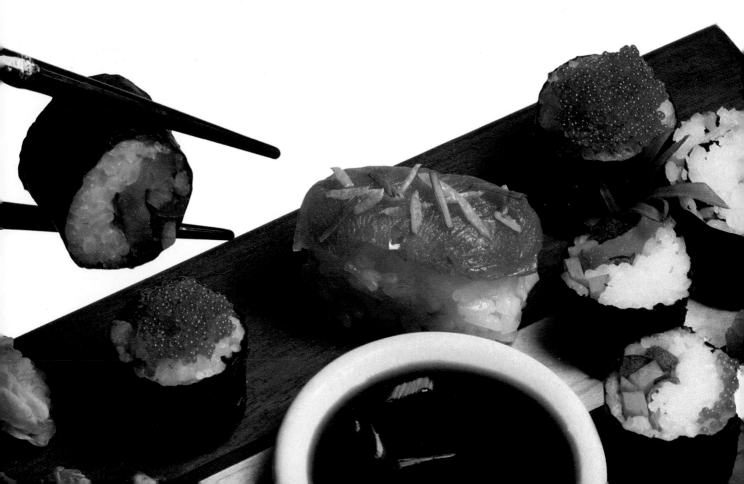

WHAT YOU CAN'T SEE CAN HURT YOU

The vicious bugs that can lay waste to your digestive tract are liable to be found anywhere. They can lurk in your nose and on your skin. They prowl in soil, in water and in sewage. They infest the intestines of cattle and chicken and pigs. And—almost always—they're in the food you eat, just waiting for the right conditions so they can thrive and multiply, sending you flying to the nearest bathroom.

They've got names like *Staphylococcus aureus*, salmonella, and *Clostridium perfringens* (the three most common causes of food poisoning in this country). There's also *Bacillus cereus, E. coli,* Vibrio, *Campylobacter jejuni* and the deadly *Clostridium botulinum.* These villainous vermin have dozens of cousins, and if a family of them jumps onto your dinner plate, it may do so in great numbers—sometimes *millions* per forkful.

With those kinds of odds, how do you come out on top, short of giving up food? The next time you enter your kitchen, should you do so screaming at the top of your lungs, carrying a knife in your teeth and spraying everything in sight with fire, buckshot and antibacterial disinfectant? Not exactly. Instead of thinking of yourself as Betty Crocker and Rambo rolled into one, consider this. The best weapons against food contaminants, say the experts, are very

Although millions of American *sushi* lovers safely enjoy raw seafood wrapped in rice and seaweed, infection experts say there's a slight chance of ingesting harmful bacteria or parasites.

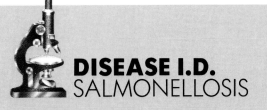

DISEASE I.D.
SALMONELLOSIS

DESCRIPTION: The almost omnipresent bacteria known as salmonella are responsible for this quite unpleasant but typically not very serious affliction. The main symptom is diarrhea, often accompanied by abdominal cramps, nausea, headache, vomiting and fever. Salmonellosis can be fatal to infants, the elderly and the already infirm.

INCIDENCE: Salmonellosis is one of the most common forms of food poisoning in the United States. Estimates of the number of cases a year have gone as high as four million. There are roughly 500 deaths annually.

MODES OF TRANSMISSION: Salmonella bacteria thrive in cooked foods such as meats, eggs and custards that have been left out of the refrigerator for several hours. These little troublemakers just love dirty utensils, greasy cutting boards, grimy tabletops and unwashed hands.

DEFENSE FACTORS: Cook all meats thoroughly. Refrigerate your leftovers as quickly as you can, and reheat them well when you're ready to eat them. Do your cooking in a scrupulously clean kitchen with scrupulously clean hands. Keep flies, roaches and rodents *far* away from food.

TREATMENT: If you have diarrhea for more than two or three days, see your physician. Antibiotic medications can be used to clear your system of the bacteria. Scientists are fearful, however, that the bacteria may grow increasingly resistant to the effects of such medications.

RECOVERY TIME: Most symptoms will disappear in two to three days.

simple. They are: soap and water, your oven, your refrigerator and a tad of common sense.

HOW TO PLAY IT SAFE

There are a number of ways in which enemy microorganisms can get into your food and grow, according to Frank Bryan, Ph.D., a food safety consultant to the World Health Organization and several large food companies. The most common are improper refrigeration, inadequate cooking and sloppy handling. Dr. Bryan suggests the following battle strategies to ensure that your next meal won't be your gastrointestinal downfall.

Refrigerate foods soon after they're cooked, unless they're kept hot. Most microorganisms don't go in much for winter sports. They'd much rather spend Christmas in a nice warm turkey breast than suffer the chills of your refrigerator. Turkey is a particularly popular hangout for bacteria because of its accommodating size, which can trap the inner warmth for hours, even in the coldest refrigerator. Cut your turkey and beef roast into pieces no thicker than 4 inches before popping them in the fridge. Apply the 4-inch rule to stacks of thinly sliced meat as well.

Make sure foods "on hold" are kept hot. So-called heat-holders, like steam tables or ovens set at low temperatures, are actually more like *warmth-holders*—and you know how fond germs are of warmth. If the internal temperature of a turkey, beef roast or other meat dish cannot be maintained at 130°F or higher, the meat shouldn't be kept warm at all.

Meats should be well cooked. The French have their *steak tartare,* but raw beef can be a raw deal when it comes to your health. Raw meat may host a number of perilous pests, like bacteria and parasitic worms, that would normally be wiped out by the heat of cooking. In addition, the FDA reports that since sushi has become popular in this country in recent years, there has been a "noticeable increase" in fish-related parasitic illness. The agency recently issued a warning that fish intended for raw con-

sumption should first be blast-frozen. (Freezing won't save you from rampant bacteria, but it can at least control the parasites.)

Don't play chicken with poultry. Be particularly careful to fully cook chicken, as about 35 percent of birds sold in this country carry salmonella bacteria. These cause salmonellosis, one of the most common food-borne illnesses in America. (As many as four million cases may occur annually.) It is largely avoidable, with proper cooking.

Reheat foods well. From the time that 25-pound turkey was first cooked to the time the last wing disappears, it's been yanked out of and shoved back into the fridge a dozen times. Each time it sits out, new microscopic hordes may have invaded. Make sure you heat that wing to at least 165°F to kill those little gremlins.

Wash your hands before handling foods. Like it or not, you could be carrying armies of the enemy germs on your hands. Be particularly careful about washing with soap and warm water after using the toilet. Human waste carries large numbers of dangerous bacteria. Open sores can also carry bacteria; if you have any on your hands, it's best to wear disposable plastic gloves.

Use clean utensils and cutting boards. A common cause of food contamination is using the same knife and cutting surface for both raw meat and fruits and vegetables. Remember that the meat will then be cooked, but the produce may not be. So don't let any dangerous hitchhikers pass from one to the other. The best thing to do is always use one cutting board for raw meats and another for other foods.

Treat beans and rice with respect. Meats aren't the only potential carriers of dangerous microorganisms. Some beans, such as black beans and pinto beans, are subject to soil contamination. So is rice. Do not let either sit overnight unrefrigerated after cooking.

And here's another tip from the FDA: Scrub your veggies, at least all those that you intend to eat raw. This is a good way to reduce the number of

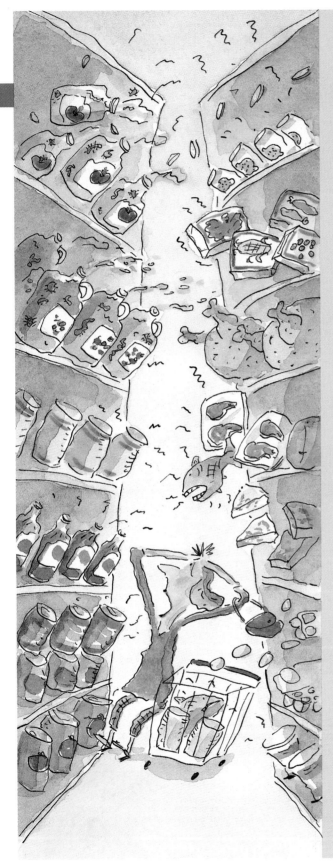

SIGNS THAT SAY "BAD FOOD"

Walking down the fluorescent-lit, linoleum-tiled aisles of your favorite supermarket, you'll see one sign for "Beverages," another for "Dairy Foods," and, of course, a sign for "Fruits." What you *won't* see are any signs that read "Bad Food—Here!"

But supermarkets from Boston to Beverly Hills occasionally do sell food that has gone bad—food that can do you and your family harm. Below, Howard Bauman, Ph.D., vice president for science and regulatory affairs with the Pillsbury Company, tells you exactly where the "bad food" markers *ought* to be placed.

Swollen cans. "Don't buy them," says Dr. Bauman. The deadly *Clostridium botulinum* bacteria may be lurking within. Carbonated beverages are an important exception to this rule—soda and beer cans often do appear slightly swollen. This is natural.

Dented cans. Some supermarkets sell them at discount prices. Buying one, says Dr. Bauman, "is a big mistake." The canning process vacuum seals foods. If the vacuum seal is broken, says Dr. Bauman, "anything can get in."

Jars with popped tops. Many glass jars today have little buttons on the lids. They should be slightly sunk into the lid. "If you can feel the button sticking out, don't buy the jar," says Dr. Bauman. If there is no pop top, then check the lid itself—it should be slightly concave. You can also listen for the hiss of air being sucked in when you open the jar at home. The hiss means it's okay.

Tampered products. Look for any signs that a product may have been opened before. Make sure, if there's a cellophane overwrap, that the wrap is intact. Some jars have heat-sealed bands. As a rule of thumb, says Dr. Bauman "compare the product to others on the shelf."

Moldy baked goods. Green and black growths on bread, rolls or cakes are a sign of trouble.

Old expiration dates. If you're buying a perishable, like milk or yogurt, the product will be marked with a last day of purchase. "I wouldn't keep it much beyond a week after that," says Dr. Bauman.

troublesome bacteria that may have jumped onto your food, either from the soil in the field or from the bin in the grocery store.

RESTAURANT SELF-DEFENSE

You can keep your own kitchen in tip-top shape, but when you decide to dine out, you give up control over how your food is handled. But there's still much you can do to protect yourself outside of the home, says Melvin N. Kramer, Ph.D., an environmental and infectious disease epidemiologist who is president of the Baltimore-based consulting firm Environmental Health Associates.

Hot foods should be hot, cold foods should be cold. "This is the cornerstone" of dining out self-defense, says Dr. Kramer. Either a hot food that's

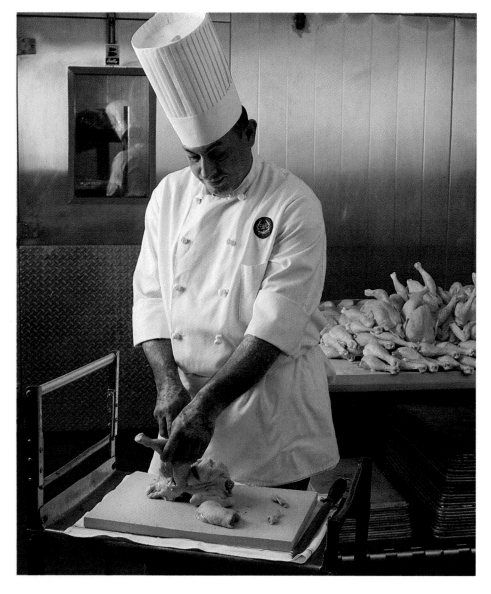

Nasty salmonella bacteria will probably never make it to the dinner plate at New York's famous Waldorf-Astoria Hotel. This air-conditioned room serves no purpose other than the preparation of raw poultry, which can harbor salmonella. Every afternoon it is scrubbed from top to bottom with water and bleach. It's *clean.*

cooled to below 140°F or a cold food that's warmed to above 45°F can get you into big trouble. If you come across a warm shrimp salad or a cool lobster thermidor, "send it back every time," says Dr. Kramer.

At salad bars, the tongs are critical. Some restaurants like to use small tongs on the theory that customers will take smaller portions. The problem with finger-sized tongs, says Dr. Kramer, is that they inevitably get dropped—finger-smudged handles and all—into the food dishes, possibly spreading disease.

What you see is what you get. Roaches scurrying along the floor? Flies buzzing around the pastry cart? "Run out of there," says Dr. Kramer. Both flies and roaches are excellent germ-carriers.

Remember that restaurant records are public records. If you want to know the hygienic track record of a certain restaurant, you can call your local health department. In some states, the restaurant must publicly post its latest inspection rating.

HIGH-TECH FOOD POISONING

While there's reason to be wise when selecting food in a restaurant, there may be just as good a reason to do the same almost anywhere. The National Research Council says residues of potentially cancer-causing pesticides on American food crops warrant concern. Scrubbing your produce with a firm brush will help to remove some of those residues.

Pesticide residues aren't the only product of the 20th century that can harm you and your immune system. Allan Johnson, coordinator of the Ontario Ministry of the Environment's Sport Fish Contaminants Program, says some North American lakes and rivers are badly polluted with highly toxic by-products of industry, such as PCBs and dioxin. These, he explains, may have been absorbed into the fish you plan to eat for dinner tonight.

As a precaution, says Johnson, you should always check with your local environmental or health agency when choosing a fishing hole. And when going to market, says Johnson, "buy from someone you can trust."

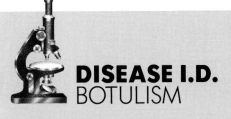

DISEASE I.D.
BOTULISM

DESCRIPTION: A type of food poisoning caused when *Clostridium botulinum* bacteria produce a toxin that thrives without air (in cans, for instance). Sufferers of botulism may experience abdominal pain, vomiting, blurred vision, muscle weakness, difficulty in breathing and swallowing and eventual paralysis. Botulism can be fatal.

INCIDENCE: Quite rare. In the United States, it is estimated that perhaps 700 people have died of botulism since 1925.

MODES OF TRANSMISSION: Most cases of botulism in this country have resulted from improper home canning of low-acid foods, such as green beans, mushrooms, spinach, olives, beef and fish. (Acid foods like tomatoes usually aren't a problem.) Commercially canned products can also carry the bacteria, but this is extremely rare.

DEFENSE FACTORS: Inspect all cans before opening. Avoid those with bulges or leaky seals. Can at home only if you are thoroughly versed in the proper techniques, and follow directions carefully.

TREATMENT: If you experience *any* of the possible signs of botulism—double or blurred vision, inability to swallow, speech or breathing difficulty—*seek immediate medical care*. Hospitalization is always required. Symptoms may appear within 12 to 36 hours after eating contaminated food.

RECOVERY TIME: If you get to a hospital quickly enough, your chances of survival are about 90 percent. Residual weakness may last for up to a year.

HEREDITY

It's hard to like a man like Herman McEllroy. Everyone knows him. Or someone just like him. He breaks all the laws of healthy living and gets away with it.

He's the one who has doughnuts for breakfast, two martinis for lunch and anything he pleases for dinner. He doesn't get enough sleep. He drinks. He smokes. And he never gets sick. He's the one whom journalists gather to interview on his 103rd birthday, and he sagely chuckles out his secret of longevity: "Good whiskey, young women and two Havana cigars a day."

Herman makes for good newspaper copy, but he's wrong about why he's lived so long.

Herman is special. When the hand was dealt in the card game of life, Herman drew a royal flush. He inherited a super immune system.

"Of course, your genetic makeup really does control everything. There are people who inherit these terrific immune systems even though they abuse them. They drink and smoke and they stay up late and they never catch anything. They go through life feeling terrific," says Terry Phillips, Ph.D., associate professor of medicine and director of the Immunogenetics and Immunochemistry Laboratories at George Washington University Medical Center.

"The genetic codes of your parents and your grandparents and your great-grandparents really do lay down the foundation of your basic immune system before you abuse it with your particular lifestyle. Some of them are so good that they can just survive anything. Others cannot," says Dr. Phillips.

So, what does it mean to inherit a "good" immune system?

Whether you were born a boy or a girl is controlled by one *single* gene. Ditto for blue eyes or brown. But your immune system involves *hundreds* of genes. Hundreds of these biological coding units of life must come together and click into place before your immune system is set up for basic functioning. It's that complex.

"We're really talking about at least two to four genes for every immunoglobulin [a type of antibody], and there are at least 5 different types of immunoglobulins. Plus we've got to get all the 10 or 12 different subtypes of cells," says Dr. Phillips, who is also the coauthor of *Winning the War Within: Understanding, Protecting, and Building Your Body's Immunity.*

"You have to think of these things as layer on layer of defense. The immune system is layers on layers and it really is designed so that if one is at fault, then another layer picks up."

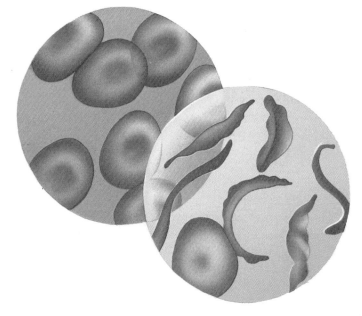

Sickle cell anemia is the result of an evolutionary experiment that didn't work. It is a genetic mutation that provides immunity against malaria, a serious infectious illness caused by a parasite that hides inside red blood cells in order to elude the body's immune defenses. The parasite can't get inside the misshapen blood cells of someone suffering from sickle cell anemia. But the price paid for such protection is too high. Many suffering from the disease experience severe symptoms and a shortened life span. (The cells at left are shaped normally, while the cells at right are the abnormal, sickle-shaped cells.)

DEFECTIVE GENES

When anything is that complex, things can go wrong. And things *do* go wrong. Sometimes children are born with immunodeficiencies. They're born without a thymus or born without any regulatory functions for the B-cells (important cellular components of the immune system), explains Dr. Phillips. Or they're born with no B-cells or antibodies. Just about every component of the immune system can be lacking at birth, and this lack is a genetic defect.

Sometimes the birth defects are so serious the child dies, as did the famous Bubble Boy who was born with no immune system at all. Other children spend the first few years of their lives receiving a battery of shots because they don't produce enough antibodies to protect them from a host of viruses that wouldn't bother anyone else.

It's also possible to inherit an immune system that's a little *too* enthusiastic. That's what happens to children who suffer from allergies.

The infant who can't stomach cow's milk, for instance, drew a gene or two that supercharges the immune system so that it thinks cow's milk is a foreign substance to be driven out of the body. Adults with allergies are in the same boat. If you can't eat clams because they make you deathly ill, you can maybe thank a great-great-grandmother back in Sweden. If it's any consolation, shellfish made her sick, too."

THROUGH THE LOOKING GLASS

Geneticists and immunogeneticists are still in the process of mapping out the human genetic code.

"If you look at a ladder that's about 100 steps high, the top of it being total knowledge of the human gene and how it works and what it does, we're probably on about rung 10 or 12," says Dr. Phillips. So what does the future hold for genetics?

"It would be nice to be able to look at cells from a pregnant woman, be able to see possible defects in the immune system and do some sort of intervention so that the infant can self-correct. It's dreaming, but it is possible," he says.

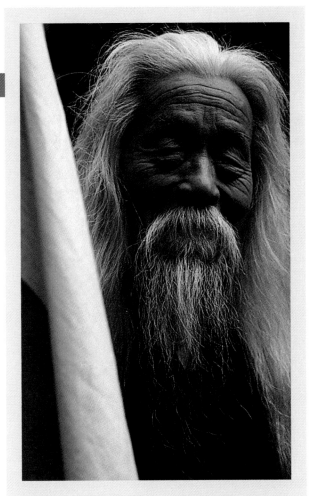

THE SECRET OF LONGEVITY

Long life. It's the elusive dream.

How do they manage it, those elders who go on and on for more than 100 birthdays?

Perhaps they do it with genes. At least in Japan they do. A Japanese study examined blood from Okinawan-Japanese nonagenarians (ages 90 to 99) and centenarians (ages 100 and over). Compared to healthy adults of all ages, researchers found that these people had an increased frequency of HLA-DR1 and an extremely low frequency of HLA-DRw9, two types of genetic "markers." The opposite configuration, high HLA-DRw9 and low HLA-DR1, is associated with susceptibility to autoimmune or immune deficiency diseases.

It seems that when nature dials in the winning genetic combination, your grand prize may be longevity.

HOME

ome, they say, is where the heart is. It's where the germs are, too. Zillions of bacteria and viruses, not to mention sundry other microscopic intruders like molds and mites splashing in your sink, lurking in your laundry, cavorting in your closets and otherwise taking up residence in more nooks and crannies than you knew your house had. Well-insulated from inclement weather and filled to the rafters with the kinds of goodies germs crave, your domicile is a dream house for microbes.

But bad as this may sound, don't dwell on it. For one thing, most of these intruders don't have killer instincts. At worst, they're merely irritating. For another, just knowing where they like to hang out and what precautions you can take to boot them out—or at least keep their numbers down—should suffice as infection protection.

Plan your strategy with this germ's-eye tour of your home.

THE WET SET

There's nothing mold spores love more than a warm, dark, damp climate like your bathroom. On the surface—and that's where you usually find it—mold

seems to pose no great threat. But some molds release toxic substances. And a good many people have allergic reactions—headaches, eye and nose irritation, sneezing, rashes, even nausea—to the spores that mold sends floating through the air. Even if you aren't allergic today, inhaling those spores could give you a problem tomorrow.

Hunt for this grayish glop at the rear base of the toilet, on the shower curtain, in the grout between ceramic tiles and in the caulking between the bathtub and wall. To get rid of it, mix vinegar and borax—a natural antimold agent—in a spray bottle. Mist the mold and wipe it off. Scrub stubborn stains with a vegetable brush. To prevent mold, keep your indoor humidity between 40 and 60 percent and sprinkle borax in corners and wherever else mold's frequently found (but not where children or pets might swallow it).

Bacteria, too, bathe in the comfort of your bathroom. The germs left after a shower or hand washing aren't in any hurry to go someplace else. Disinfect your sink, tub and toilet—don't just wash them with water—about once a week, says Beth Whitman, a Pennsylvania State University home economist.

TOSS THAT TOOTHBRUSH

Using the same old toothbrush month after month could take a bite out of your health, say researchers at the University of Oklahoma.

Because toothbrushes bristle with bacteria, people suffering from oral infections may get better faster if they start using a new brush every two weeks.

But an aging toothbrush might expose anyone to problems. Natural bristles, especially, draw water and bacteria into their hollow cores. But germs can inhabit synthetics, too.

Your toothbrush can become contaminated as quickly as a week after its initial use. Replace it at least once a month, and right away after any illness.

HEALTHY HOUSEHOLD HUMIDITY

Note: Decrease in bar width indicates decrease in danger		Optimum Zone	
Bacteria			
Viruses			
Fungi			
Mites			
Respiratory infections*			
Allergic rhinitis and asthma			
Chemical interactions			
Ozone production			
*Insufficient data above 50 percent relative humidity	10 20 30 40 50 60 70 80 90 Relative Humidity (%)		

Reprinted by permission of the American Society of Heating, Refrigerating and Air-Conditioning Engineers, Inc., Atlanta, Ga. from *ASHRAE Transactions 1985*, vol. 91, part 1B.

Improper humidity levels in your home can put a damper on health. Low humidity dries out the infection-resistant membranes of your nose and throat. High humidity spawns the growth of allergy-provoking fungi and dust mites. Keep humidity between 40 and 60 percent for fewer problems.

If you're living it up with a home hot tub or whirlpool, be advised that bubbling bacteria have been linked to skin rashes and other ills, including Legionnaires' disease. Make sure you follow the manufacturer's sanitation recommendations.

EVERYTHING PLUS THE KITCHEN SINK

Commonsense measures are generally adequate to keep your kitchen clean of unwanted organisms, says Gerald Kuhn, Ph.D., professor of food science at Pennsylvania State University. But one person's common sense might be another's common error. Here are the basics.

Wooden cutting boards. Bacteria-laden particles from food you are preparing, along with mold, sneak into cut marks and are absorbed into pores in the wood, where they wait to contaminate other food later, says Dr. Kuhn. Wash cutting boards with detergent and warm water, then rinse. For extra protection, prepare a solution of one part bleach (5 percent laundry bleach) and eight parts water. Spread it over the board and let it evaporate. Scrub the board from time to time with fine sandpaper to reduce the size of its absorbent pores. The same instructions go for wooden utensils. Better yet, use ones made of plastic or stainless steel.

Sponges. Using a sponge to wash your dishes and wipe up spills, greasy fingerprints and who knows what else is "bad news," says Dr. Kuhn. "Sponges absorb food and serve as incubators for germs." Instead, use dishcloths that are laundered on a regular basis.

Sink. Look for mold between the sink and the wall and around the bottom of the cold water pipe. Banish it with the same vinegar/borax mixture previously prescribed for in your bathroom.

Refrigerator. Temperatures vary throughout your refrigerator. Areas above 40°F attract mold, which can contaminate your food with toxins. Wash it off refrigerator surfaces and then apply disinfectant. Disinfect your entire refrigerator about once a month. This goes for self-defrosting refrigerators, too. And clean mold out of the surplus-water tray (reach along the bottom of the refrigerator to see if you have one) and then sprinkle the dry surface with borax.

Stove. Bacteria in your oven are baked to death every time you fire it up, but stove vents can clog up with mold and bacteria, so clean them regularly.

Garbage. Keep it covered so it doesn't attract flies and other disease-carrying insects. And sprinkle the bottom of the garbage pail with borax or baking soda to prevent mold.

CELLAR SENSE

Mold may be happy to lounge in your bathroom, but in your basement, it's more productive. "Most

(continued on page 44)

HOME HOT SPOTS

From attic to cellar, your home is rife with energetic life forms, most of them not your family's. Fortunately, they don't usually have the ability or inclination to do serious damage to their human hosts. After all, without you, where would they be? Certainly not making themselves at home with the cozy comforts your place offers. Here are some of their favorite spots.

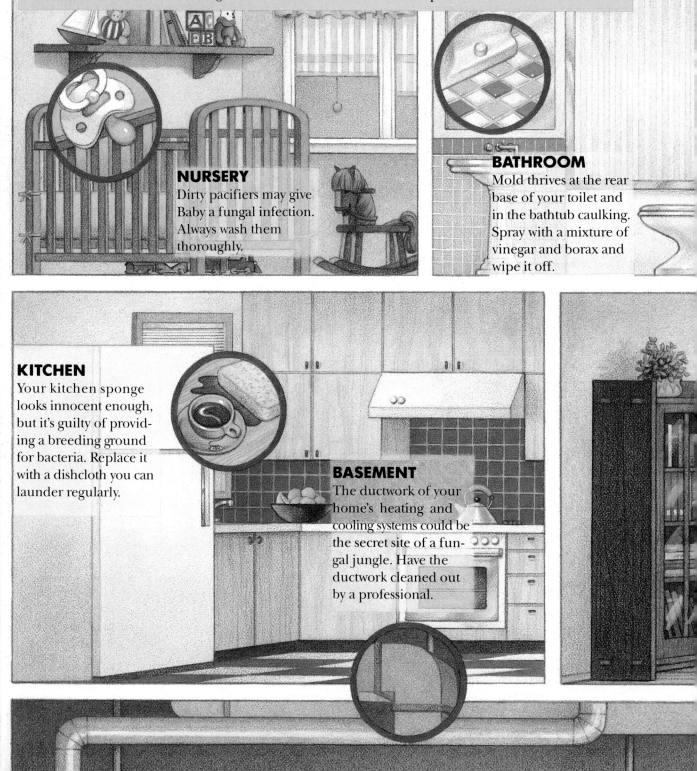

NURSERY
Dirty pacifiers may give Baby a fungal infection. Always wash them thoroughly.

BATHROOM
Mold thrives at the rear base of your toilet and in the bathtub caulking. Spray with a mixture of vinegar and borax and wipe it off.

KITCHEN
Your kitchen sponge looks innocent enough, but it's guilty of providing a breeding ground for bacteria. Replace it with a dishcloth you can launder regularly.

BASEMENT
The ductwork of your home's heating and cooling systems could be the secret site of a fungal jungle. Have the ductwork cleaned out by a professional.

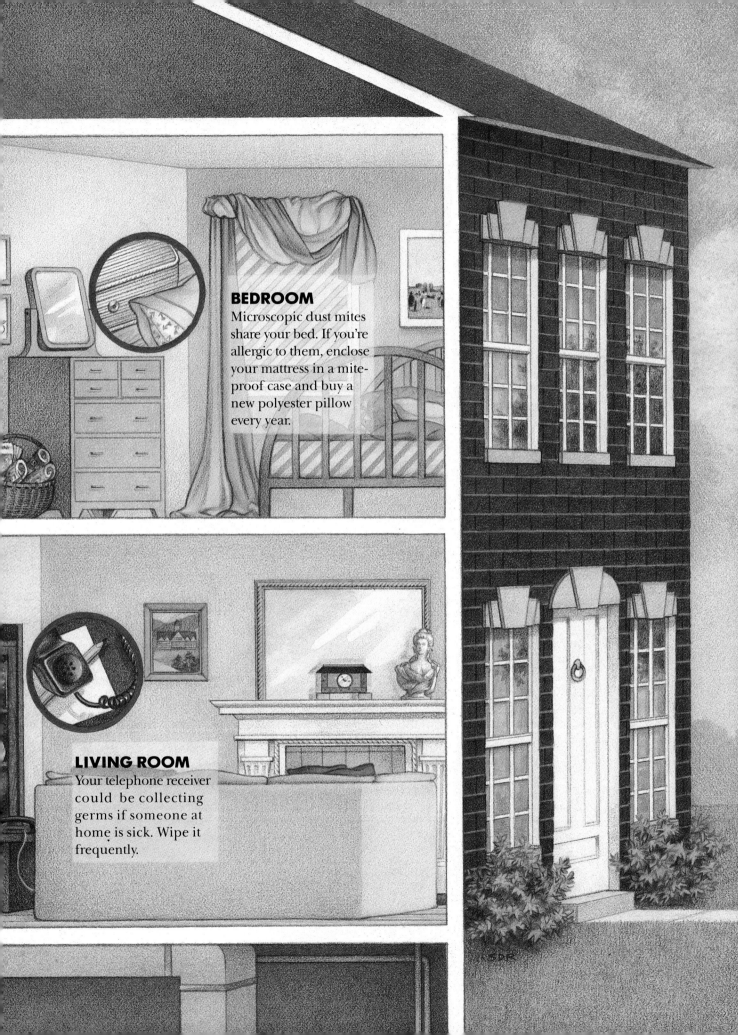

BEDROOM
Microscopic dust mites share your bed. If you're allergic to them, enclose your mattress in a mite-proof case and buy a new polyester pillow every year.

LIVING ROOM
Your telephone receiver could be collecting germs if someone at home is sick. Wipe it frequently.

basements are at least a little damp, and most produce mold spores by the millions that gradually float upstairs to waft through the house," notes Alfred Zamm, M.D., author of *Why Your House May Endanger Your Health.*

Potential hideouts for mold are your basement walls and piles of old newspapers and clothes in your laundry area. The ductwork in your heating and air-conditioning systems could also be creeping with a jungle of fungus. To combat these intruders, make your basement as dry as possible by patching cracks and installing a dehumidifier. Wash your clothes, trash your junk and call a professional to clean out your air vents.

NURSERY RHYME REALITY

Hickory, dickory, dock. The germs stay round the clock. Infants, with their not-well-developed immune systems, are more susceptible than adults to infectious diseases. And the nursery is crawling with potential for infection.

Common sense suggests that you promptly dispose of dirty diapers and keep surfaces all squeaky clean.

If your baby's pacifier is dirty, he could develop an ugly fungal infection of the mouth called thrush. Always thoroughly clean pacifiers with soap and water and have several on hand so the one in his mouth is clean.

DETOXIFY YOUR HOUSEHOLD CLEANERS

Unlike Grandma, who used lots of soapy water for her housecleaning, the modern homemaker can choose from a vast array of chemicals for everything from wiping off grease to wiping out germs. But some of these powerful substances might have toxic effects. If you're looking for a better solution, try these.

SUBSTANCE	TOXIC EFFECTS	SYMPTOMS	ALTERNATIVES
Oven and drain cleaners	Highly corrosive, they can cause severe skin and eye damage.	Cleaners cause rapidly formed chemical burns that are slow to heal.	Oven cleaners: Use baking soda for scouring. For baked-on grease, put ¼ cup ammonia in oven overnight to loosen, scrub with baking soda. Drain cleaners: Pour ½ cup salt down drain followed by boiling water; flush with hot tap water.
Wall and floor cleaners	All toxic, especially cleaners containing petroleum distillates.	Diethylene glycol depresses the central nervous system and causes liver and kidney changes.	Use dishwashing liquid for large areas, rinse if necessary.
Toilet bowl cleaners	Those containing acid or bleaches are corrosive.	Bleach cleaners cause chemical burns that are slow to heal. Acid cleaners cause ulceration and chemical burns.	For light stains, mix borax and lemon juice into a paste. After flushing, rub on paste, let set 2 hours before scrubbing.
Disinfectants	Toxic, corrosive.	Phenol (carbolic acid) causes chemical burns, can be absorbed through the skin.	Rubbing alcohol, soap or detergent. Avoid products containing phenol or cresol.

SCENT-SITIVITY

Someone sent you that beautiful bouquet of flowers on your living room table? How sweet it is—unless you happen to suffer from bronchial asthma or hay fever. In that case, a deep whiff could leave you wheezing or sneezing, warns a study by a group of Swedish researchers.

For some sufferers, the problem stems from an allergy to the flowers' pollen, they say. For others, odorants or irritants originating from the flowers bring on the symptoms. Flowers with strong scents are most likely to produce symptoms.

Commenting on the Swedish study, Harold Nelson, M.D., chief of adult allergy at the National Jewish Center for Immunology and Respiratory Medicine in Denver, says that pollen from flowers rarely presents a problem for his asthma patients. "But odors certainly can be primary irritants. Christmas trees, which probably release a lot of resins into the air, are a good example of that. When people bring them into their homes, their asthma gets worse."

People with asthma have what is called twitchy lungs. All of us have nerve cells called irritant receptors in our lungs that react to and protect us against foreign substances in the air, Dr. Nelson explains. But the irritant receptors in the lungs of asthmatics overreact, leaving their victims gasping for breath.

If you're a hay fever sufferer, flowers could bring into full bloom your familiar symptoms of frequent sneezing, runny nose and red, watery, itchy eyes.

Steer your nose clear of strong-smelling flowers such as hyacinths, lilies of the valley, lilacs, chrysanthemums, marigolds and daffodils. You'll breathe easier if you don't wear perfume or colognes, either. And ask friends to leave their bottled scents behind when they visit.

Researchers have found bacteria that cause infant rashes, ear infections and pneumonia in the residual dampness in those thick sponges used to cradle babies during their baths. Make sure your child's sponge dries thoroughly between uses. If you're not sure, throw it in the clothes dryer.

BEDDING DOWN

The variety of fabrics in your bedroom offers attractions aplenty for dust mites—tiny insects that thrive in even the cleanest of homes—especially in the bedroom. They can cause sneezing, congestion, watery eyes and skin problems—allergic reactions not to the mites themselves (they don't come onto your skin at all) but to their feces.

Mites feast on the tiny flakes of old skin you and your loved ones constantly shed. Furniture and carpets are popular eating spots, but your mattress is a virtual 24-hour diner. If mite allergies give you trouble, enclose your mattress in a mite-proof case, wash your bedding frequently and purchase a new polyester pillow every year.

Mold, that old hanger-on, loves your bedroom clothes closet. Keep mold under wraps by installing a louvered closet door to increase air circulation.

The bedroom is Infection Central when someone is sick in bed. Colds and the flu are easily transmitted via doorknobs and even the telephone receiver.

CLEAN LIVING

A big problem in the living room is dust, which contains those nasty dust mites. If they cause problems for you, consider replacing your wall-to-wall carpeting with smaller rugs that you can clean outside.

Do all your indoor cleaning with damp, not dry, mops and dust rags, says Whitman. Otherwise, you're just moving the dust from one spot to another. And make sure your vacuum cleaner is clean, or it will be spewing out more dust than it's sucking up.

HOSPITALS

If you were a patient admitted to the typical hospital of 135 years ago, you would have been horrified. Hospital walls and ceilings then, wrote Florence Nightingale, were "saturated with impurity" and often streamed with moisture until "a minute vegetation appeared." The odor, she said, was "sickening." Not surprisingly, Nightingale maintained that your chances of surviving illness were better at home.

Things have improved a lot since then. The typical modern American hospital is a glistening, ultra-sanitized, glass-and-chrome, high-tech bastion of (seemingly) bacteria-free purity. It's an apparently well-run, well-maintained institution where sick people lumber in and healthy people bounce out. You might think it very unlikely that anyone would contract an infection in such an environment.

Yet it happens. Doctors even have a fancy term for infections picked up during a hospital stay: nosocomial infections.

Wes W., a 29-year-old Maryland man, got a doozy of one. He checked into a classy private hospital with a minor nasal obstruction and wound up with a nasty infection that devoured most of the cartilage in his nose. Marguerite T., in Michigan, checked in for a gallbladder operation, and a gangrenous infection saw to it that she wouldn't check out for 38 days. Reid C., a Pennsylvania high school student, had a touch of viral pneumonia that brought him into a hospital. While there, he contracted a more serious bacterial infection that required surgical scraping of his lung.

Wes, Marguerite and Reid are *far* from alone. Government experts and others estimate that from 5 to 10 percent or more of all people checking into American hospitals fall victim to infections that are wholly unrelated to the illnesses for which they were admitted. "It's no joke. We have a real problem in our hospitals," says Lowell S. Levin, Ed.D., professor of public health at Yale University's School of Medicine.

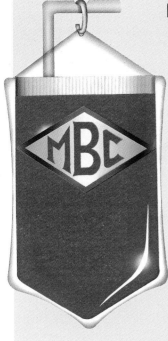

BE YOUR OWN BLOOD DONOR

Fill out the forms. Roll up your sleeve. Lie down. "We'll just tighten this tourniquet a bit." Clench your fist. Look away. It's time to donate blood.

Altruistic reasons aside, donating blood may reduce your own risk of infection the next time you plan a hospital visit.

The best of all times to donate your own blood to be used for yourself is when you're scheduled for surgery, says Ralph L. Bernstein, M.D., chairman of the Department of Anesthesiology at New York's Hospital for Joint Diseases Orthopedic Institute and associate professor of anesthesiology at Mount Sinai School of Medicine. "You give blood now, then you get it back when you need it so you don't have to expose yourself to the possibility of getting blood that has hepatitis, AIDS or other infections in it."

How common are such infections? Not very, at least now that all hospitals test for AIDS in blood donors. There is, however, always a small risk, says Dr. Bernstein—a risk that can be totally avoided with a preoperative donation of your own blood. "So if your surgeon says you'll need blood, donating beforehand is *absolutely* the thing to do," he says.

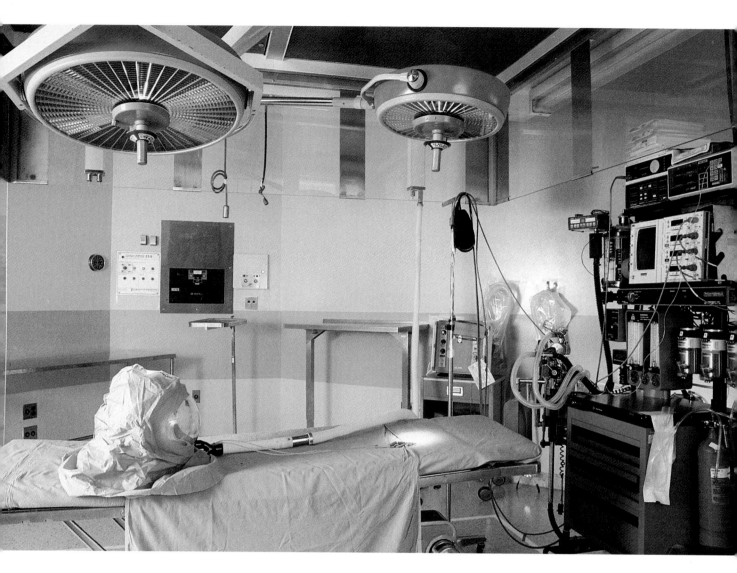

A BREEDING GROUND FOR INFECTIONS

"There's no mystery as to how these things are caused," says Dr. Levin. "You've got a large collection of sick people, some with infectious diseases, and you've got a very busy, stressed staff." If the staff cuts corners— not washing their hands or not sterilizing equipment— "they can flit around like bumblebees spreading infection from patient to patient," he says.

Barry Farr, M.D., hospital epidemiologist at the University of Virginia Medical Center, admits that unwashed hands are a contributing factor, but "the majority of infections," he says, "are caused by the patient's own flora." That is to say, bacteria that is normally present on the skin can create havoc when they get inside the body of an already weakened patient during any kind of invasive procedure.

There's clean and there's *clean*. Some hospitals today are equipped with "clean-air" operating rooms, such as this one at Philadelphia's Thomas Jefferson University Hospital. Powerful filtration systems suck out even the tiniest fleck of dirt, minimizing the risk of airborne infection. That's not a spacesuit on the table; it's a special outfit for doctors and nurses that inhibits the spread of germs.

One such procedure is the insertion of a catheter into the urinary tract. According to a study published in the *American Journal of Epidemiology*, urinary tract infections (due largely to catheter use) constitute 42 percent of all nosocomial infections. The next most common kinds are surgical wound infections (like Wes's and Marguerite's), which constitute 24 percent; and infections of the lungs (like Reid's), that make up another 10 percent.

FIGHTING BACK WHILE ON YOUR BACK

Dr. Farr and Dr. Levin agree that there are measures the patient can and should take to make sure a visit to the hospital doesn't turn into an infectious nightmare.

• "If a doctor or other health care worker comes in to work on you, politely ask if he has washed his hands," suggests Dr. Farr. If all hospital staff workers were fastidious hand-washers, the patient's risk of nosocomial infection could be cut by more than half, says Dr. Levin.

• Ask your surgeon if presurgical shaving can be avoided. Shaving you before surgery, says Dr. Levin, "is one of those knee-jerk, automatic things that are done in medical care like in anything else." For many operations, particularly gynecological ones, it just isn't necessary, he says. "Shaving makes little nicks and cuts and opens up a vast avenue for infections."

• Shop around for a hospital. Most hospitals will simply not tell you what their nosocomial infection rates are. However, "hospitals that don't have infection control programs can be expected to have higher nosocomial infection rates," says Dr. Farr. So ask if such a program exists. (For details on one hospital's program, see the box "Infection Control Coordinator: Kathy Hinkle.")

• The less time you're in the hospital, the less chance you have of picking up any loitering germs. Talk to your doctor about what you might be able to do in advance to shorten your hospital stay.

• When you speak with your doctors and nurses, show them that you are an alert and informed medical consumer, says Dr. Levin. Let them know that you are concerned about the problem of hospital infections. This simple communication, says Dr. Levin, "can make all the difference."

• Lastly, says Dr. Levin, keep in mind that many medical procedures can be done—and should be done—in a doctor's office. "Hospitals are not hotels, so don't think of them that way," he says. Opt for a hospital stay only if there are no other options.

Florence Nightingale would surely agree.

WHERE GERMS GET AN EDUCATION

Infections in large teaching hospitals are almost twice as common as in nonteaching hospitals, a government study found. Barry Farr, M.D., says however, that this doesn't mean that the larger the hospital, the dirtier. Rather, he says, sicker patients requiring more complicated medical procedures explain the difference in infection rates.

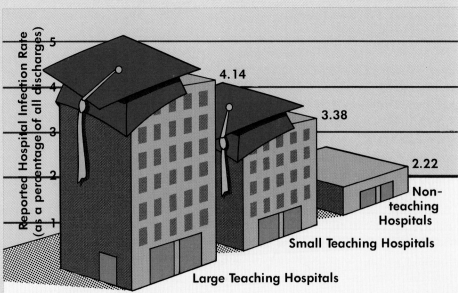

Reported Hospital Infection Rate (as a percentage of all discharges)

4.14 — Large Teaching Hospitals
3.38 — Small Teaching Hospitals
2.22 — Non-teaching Hospitals

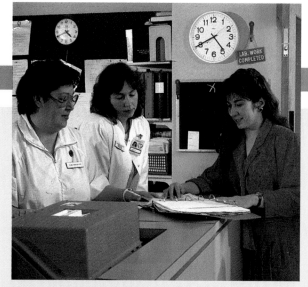

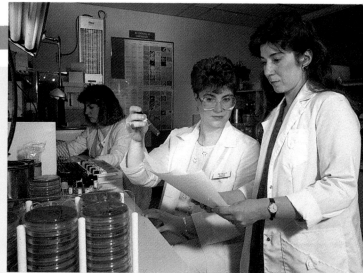

INFECTION CONTROL COORDINATOR: KATHY HINKLE

Nosocomial (hospital-spread) infections—they're nightmares for patients, and hospitals don't like them much either. But a government study in 1985 found that 32 percent of such infections could be eliminated with in-house nosocomial infection control programs.

Featured on this page (in red dress) is Kathy Hinkle, R.N., coordinator of such a program for The Medical Center at Princeton, a private New Jersey hospital. In addition to her experience as a registered nurse, she received special training at the federal Centers for Disease Control before assuming her current duties.

These duties, says Hinkle, include (clockwise from top left): working with the staff to make sure that any human errors are not repeated, reviewing infection-battling procedures taking place in the lab, monitoring hospital procedures and training new employees in infection-fighting strategies.

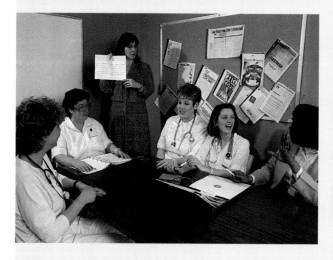

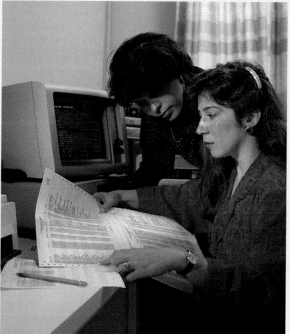

HOW YOUR IMMUNE SYSTEM WORKS

Your body declares war every day. You may be a peace-loving person, a gentle soul, a humane Mahatma Gandhi who wouldn't harm even an insect. It doesn't matter. The microscopic world is one of fight or flight—and your body knows it.

Your immune system is a superefficient war machine. It fights invaders with cellular troops willing to martyr themselves for the cause, powerful chemicals that explode or digest the enemy, and a counterintelligence department that keeps dossiers on every enemy encountered. Your immune system is on constant alert, and it is fully automatic. If this weren't so, you wouldn't be alive to read this page.

The brave little soldier cells of the immune system—that metaphor is already a cliché. But we had to trot it out yet again. There is no other way. Science writers keep *trying* to get away from martial imagery. They try, but they fail—for good reason.

"I tried desperately to get away from military terms when I wrote my book, but you have to use them. If you think of your body as a country, your immune system *is* the army," says Terry Phillips, Ph.D., associate professor of medicine and director of the Immunogenetics and Immunochemistry Laboratories at George Washington University Medical Center and coauthor of *Winning the War Within: Understanding, Protecting, and Building Your Body's Immunity.*

"It's a battlefield. Put some lymphocytes (white blood cells) and some self-respecting bacteria in a test tube and watch what happens. It's quite horrible. Those little white cells throw themselves into the battle and they give up their lives. They throw themselves in willingly to die and their whole thought, it seems, is keeping you happy. And it happens every day."

Of course, the dramatic scenario of invasion and defense doesn't usually take place in a test tube. The setting is the blood vessels, sinews and tissues of your body. And the battle is much more complex than lymphocyte versus bacterium. Lymphocytes and microbes do frequently slug it out in the hidden recesses of your body, but more than that goes on.

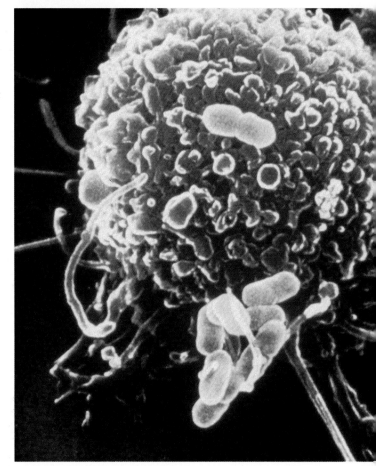

A whole lot more.

The multilayered defenses of your immune system have a kind of architecture. They fit together with the complex precision of a symphony. And, as in any other army, there are specialized units—some do the fighting, some instruct and train raw recruits, some keep records. There's even a unit that picks up and disposes of the casualties.

Come, let us journey within, to the liquid realm of what may be the most awesome fighting force on the face of the earth—your body's immune system.

THE FACE OF THE ENEMY

But wait. How can you tell an immunological warrior from a wimp if you don't get a look at the opponent?

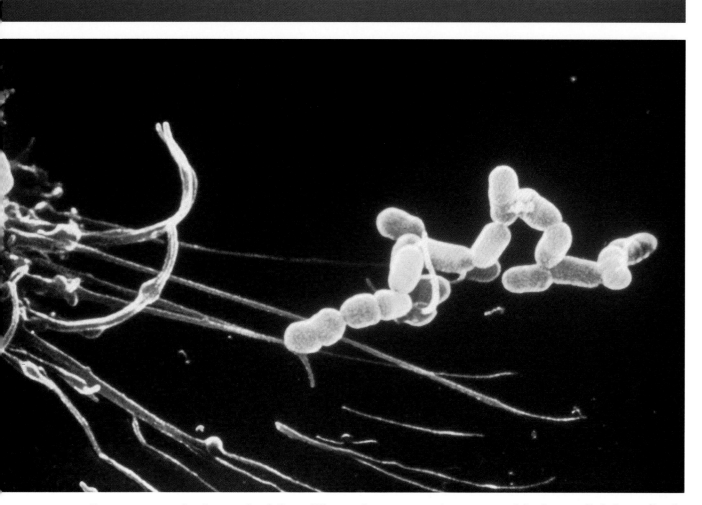

In one corner, having evolved for millions of years as a specialized fighting force, we have the human immune system. In the other corner, having evolved for millions of years in conjunction and competition with that system we have . . . the enemy.

Don't underestimate the bad guys (known as antigens)—bacteria, viruses, parasites, assorted microbes, fungi and yeasts. They may be microscopic, but they've got you surrounded. More than a million bacteria may inhabit just one square inch of your *freshly washed* skin. You scoop up germs when you play with your children or pet your puppy. They hitch a ride on your fork on the way into your mouth. They take to the air, swimming in the little water droplets expelled by your co-worker's sneeze. And when you kiss . . . let's just say that

A macrophage, one of the largest fighting cells of the immune system, lassos invading bacteria. A cell with a voracious appetite (*macro* means large and *phage* means eater), the macrophage digests its hapless victims.

you and your partner are exchanging something besides affection.

Although many microbes are harmless to humans (and some are even beneficial), there are less savory types that would like nothing better than to take up residence inside your body and raise a ruckus as well as a family—a big family. If they successfully cross the border, getting past the barriers of your skin and the mucous membranes of your respiratory, digestive and urogenital tracts, they make you sick.

(continued on page 55)

THE HUMAN DEFENSE DEPARTMENT: WHO'S ON THE JOB

Like a magnificent machine, the various parts of the immune system work together. When an invading bacterium—the hot dog–shaped object on the right—triggers the defense mechanisms of human immunity, a whole cascade of events takes place. The cells of the immune system communicate and cooperate in a wonderful harmony that usually vanquishes the foe.

The cells of the immune system are born in bone marrow. There are two general types, those for general defense (your nonspecific immune system) and those that go after special targets (your specific immune system.)

The general defense (purple area) consists of feeding cells—macrophages, granulocytes, monocytes. All the specific immune cells (turquoise area) are lymphocytes. There are two general types of lymphocytes, B-cells and T-cells.

Lymphocytes that have gone through the thymus gland come out educated as T-cells. Killer T-cells do the dirty work of killing any cells in your body that have been invaded by viruses. Helper T-cells and suppressor T-cells regulate the magnitude of the immune response and help bring things back to normal when the infection is conquered.

B-cells are lymphocytes that have been educated in the bone marrow. B-cells turn into plasma cells when they encounter foreign microbes or substances that turn them on.

Your plasma cells produce Y-shaped antibodies and your whole body produces complement; both are proteins that attach themselves to invaders. The immune system usually wins its fights quickly. When it doesn't, you're the first to know.

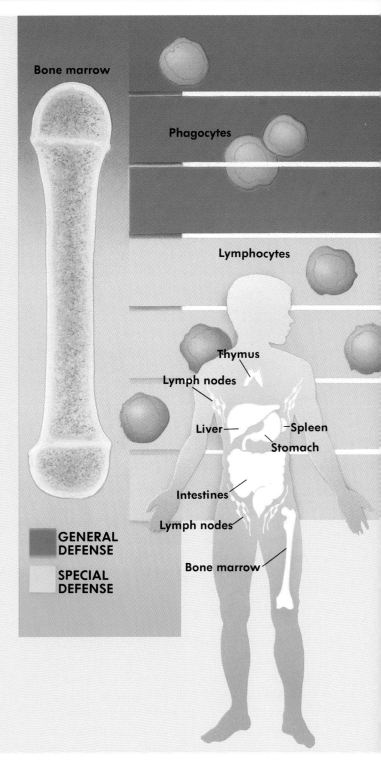

Bone marrow

Phagocytes

Lymphocytes

Thymus

Lymph nodes

Liver

Spleen

Stomach

Intestines

Lymph nodes

Bone marrow

GENERAL DEFENSE

SPECIAL DEFENSE

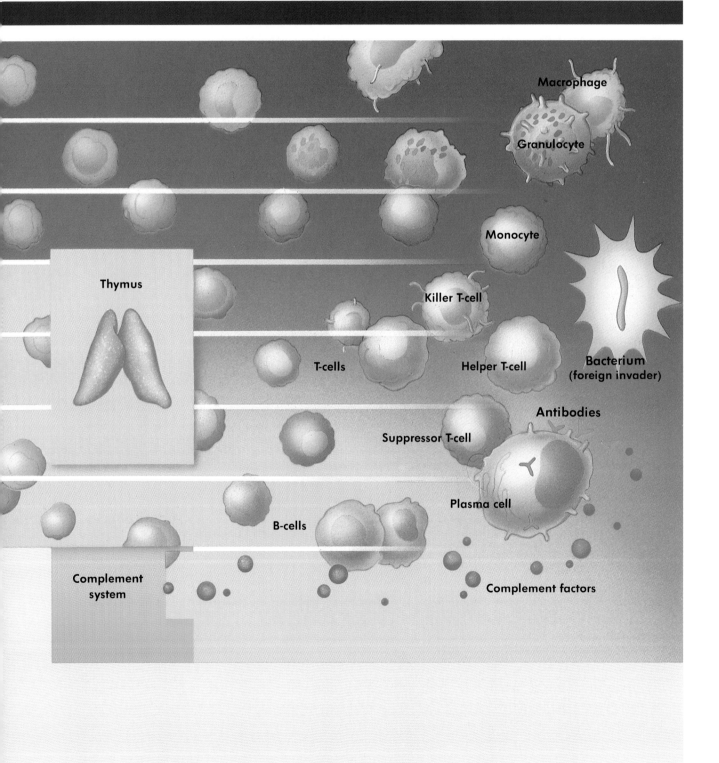

Macrophage

Granulocyte

Monocyte

Killer T-cell

Thymus

T-cells

Helper T-cell

Bacterium
(foreign invader)

Antibodies

Suppressor T-cell

Plasma cell

B-cells

Complement
system

Complement factors

KNOW YOUR ENEMIES

When you fall ill, it's usually bacteria or viruses that trip you up. What are these mysterious creatures, so small that you can't see them with the naked eye, but mighty enough to lay low the strongest human?

Although we tend to think of both bacteria and viruses as "germs," they are really very different.

Bacteria are single-celled organisms, generally rod shaped, that propel themselves about with whiplike tails known as flagella. Bacteria multi-

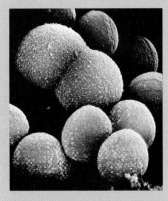

Staphylococcus is a bacterium that is especially devious in eluding the defenses of your immune system.

ply by dividing themselves. If one gets inside you and goes unchallenged, it soon becomes two, two become four, four become eight and so forth.

Many bacteria are not harmful to humans. Some, such as the ones that live in your intestines, are even good for you, helping you to digest your food. But when bacteria are bad, they can be very bad. They are the cause of such human ills as leprosy, tetanus, tuberculosis and pneumonia.

Harmful bacteria cause their damage by

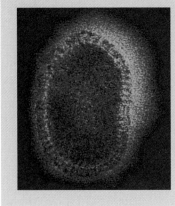

Your immune system knows the influenza virus well. There are several strains of influenza virus, and new ones develop all the time.

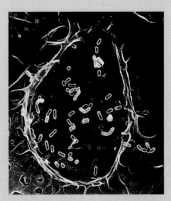

Escherichia coli, aka E. coli, are common bacteria, found in great numbers in your intestines.

excreting toxic wastes after feeding. Although some of these bacteria are really crafty and give the human immune system a merry chase, the good news is that antibiotics can stop them.

Viruses have the edge over bacteria in the smallness department. They are anywhere from 10 to 1,000 times smaller. They come in a variety of geometrical shapes. Some look like little rocket ships escaped from a science fiction

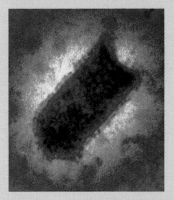

The herpes virus causes its share of human grief. The immune system keeps the virus dormant but can't kill it.

movie; others resemble miniature jewels.

Viruses, only partly alive, need *you* in order to reproduce. They slip inside the cells of your body and take over the DNA, which they use to make copies of themselves. Your cell becomes *their* nursery, from which thousands of their offspring pour out to snatch other cells.

Viruses are responsible for most diseases that are the lot of humankind. You can blame viruses for everything from influenza and the common cold to polio and some types of cancer. Although your body's immune system is equipped to deal with viruses, it must do so without outside help. Viruses cannot be controlled with antibiotics.

Successful invasions have names like polio, tuberculosis, hepatitis, influenza, the common cold. Successful invasions can also take the form of localized infections.

THIS MEANS WAR

Let's take a closer look at an infection.

You've finally gotten around to cleaning the basement. That pile of wood scraps over there has got to go, and you begin carting and hauling and . . . *ouch!* What was that? A rusty nail, and you took it in the palm? There's a dark little spot on your hand and no blood. Nasty business. Nastier, perhaps, than you realize.

Let's zero in on that puncture wound, reduce ourselves down to microscopic size and zip inside where the invasion has begun. Bacteria that rode in on the nail are already cavorting in the nice, warm nutrients provided by your blood and enjoying what they think is going to be their new home.

But their doom is already sealed. As soon as the skin was broken, a silent chemical alarm went off: *The border has been breached. Illegal aliens are swarming across. Help!*

If the bacteria could see the neutrophils headed their way in response to that alarm, they would probably trample each other in the scramble to back out of the puncture wound.

Meet the neutrophil. This cell is part of what is called your nonspecific immune system. Translated, that means it'll take on anything in sight that isn't you. Neutrophils are also one of a number of cells known as phagocytes. *Phago* means eating, and *cyte* means cell. To the "cell-eating" neutrophils, the bacteria that came through that wound might as well be orders of hamburgers and french fries as they close in rapidly for the feast.

Neutrophils might be compared to the foot soldiers of the immune system. There are a lot of them, and they're on constant border patrol just looking for invaders. They move quickly, swimming in your blood and oozing amoebalike through the walls of your blood vessels to attack on command.

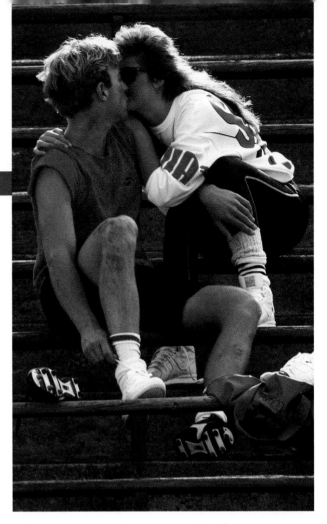

Shared intimacy also means shared germs. Everyday activities bring you in contact with untold millions of microbes, most of which never pose a problem. But fear not. Those microbes that do slip past the body's outer covering meet the multilayered defenses of the human immune system.

When the message comes that the walls of the skin have been breached, they are *there*.

THE TANKS ROLL IN

As if the invading bacteria weren't in enough trouble, behind the neutrophil comes a monster of a cell—the macrophage. Macrophages might be big compared with the other cells of your immune system and they might be slow, but they are tough.

"They could eat an infinite number of bacteria as long as they don't eat them too fast. The job turns them on," says Gary Wood, Ph.D., professor of pathology at the University of Kansas Medical Center. Dr. Wood has conducted research on macrophages for a number of years.

Macrophages tend to more or less hang around, not moving too much. But when a chemical signal brings the ruckus of an invasion to their attention, they ooze on over to see what the trouble is. Once the macrophages come upon the battle scene and get into the fray, they liven up and become more mobile, says Dr. Wood.

Like the neutrophil, the macrophage is non-specific and a phagocyte. And like the neutrophil, it flows around its prey, envelops it inside its body and secretes digestive enzymes on it. Invading bacteria experience death by digestion.

TAKE OUT THE GARBAGE, DEAR

Macrophages also do garbage detail. The specific immune system, which we'll get to shortly, is quite messy in its battles. It literally explodes the enemy, scattering bits of cellular debris.

Even before an infection is over, macrophages begin mopping up the battlefield. They "devour" the remains of invading microorganisms as well as the cellular casualties from your own immune system. They clear the battlefield of "corpses" so that life can go on.

There are also macrophages whose whole role in life consists of garbage detail. They line your lungs and eat any foreign particles that get through the filtering system of your nose. They gobble up dust, asbestos fibers, pollen and other troublemakers. If you happen to be a smoker, many of the macrophages in your lungs are black from continually lapping up tars in the smoke.

"Macrophages go around and clean up things that aren't supposed to be in the body, and then they just digest them," says Dr. Wood.

CALLING IN THE SPECIALISTS

The macrophage is bigger and slower than a neutrophil. It is also much more talented than a neutrophil, according to Michael Lieber, M.D., Ph.D., immunologist at the National Institutes of Health (NIH).

After a macrophage finishes its meal, it burps out pieces of the offending substances (antigens) and puts them out on its surface. It shows them to a different class of immune cells, known as lymphocytes.

When the lymphocytes get a look at the antigens, a whole different component of the immune system kicks in. It's almost as though the macrophage is preparing a tray of appetizers for the lymphocytes to sample.

"The macrophage is like the second in command to the lymphocytes. It's very obedient, very obsequious," says Dr. Lieber.

Before we move on to the exquisite intricacies of that other major component of our defense forces, known as the specific immune system, we need to meet one more nonspecific cell.

BENEDICT ARNOLD, BEWARE

Yet another avenger stalks through your body—the natural killer cell, alias the NK cell. This cell doesn't ambush invaders. Its mission in life is to eradicate turncoats.

Every army in the world deals harshly with traitors, and the human immune system is no exception.

The full function and abilities of the natural killer cell are far from understood, but it is revealing some of its secrets, according to John Clancy, Jr., Ph.D., head of the Department of Anatomy and Cell Biology at Loyola University Stritch School of Medicine in Maywood, Illinois.

Natural killer cells target certain types of cancer cells, which are actually your body's own cells that have begun behaving unnaturally and multiplying rapidly. Natural killer cells may also go after any of your body's cells that have been damaged by viruses, bacteria or fungi. It's still unclear exactly how they know that a cell has gone bad. There seems to be some sort of marker on the target cell's surface that betrays it, says Dr. Clancy.

When the natural killer cell comes upon another cell that is not behaving itself—a traitor, if you will—it liquidates the offender. We use the word "liquidate" advisedly. The natural killer cell attaches itself to the bad cell and secretes a protein known as perforin onto its surface. The offending cell then leaks out its contents.

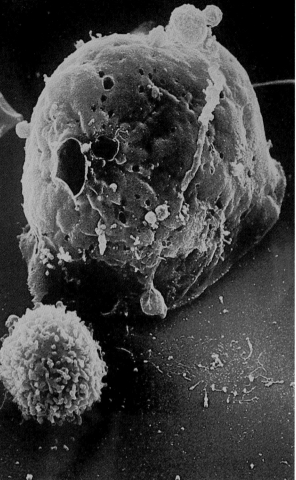

Caution, killer at work. Thank goodness. At right, a killer cell confronts a tumor cell. It kills by attaching itself to the larger tumor cell and injecting it with a chemical that perforates it, causing the contents to leak out. The photo below shows the vanquished tumor cell. All that remains is the threadlike structure that held it together.

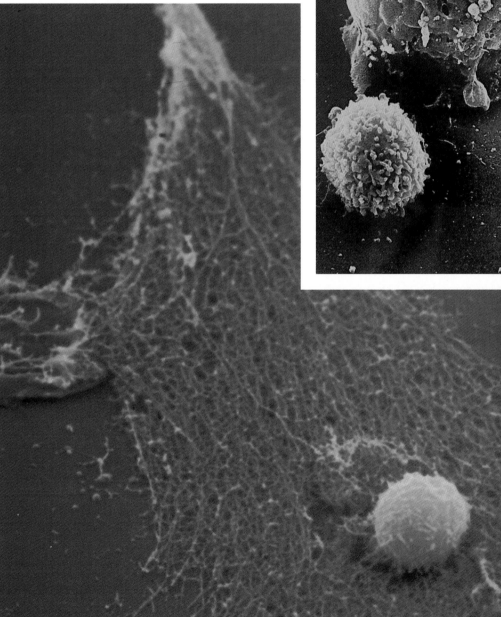

Natural killer cells are currently generating a good deal of excitement in the research community, says Dr. Clancy. Ways are being sought to rev up their cancer-fighting abilities, and results so far have been promising.

THE KILLER ELITE

Every army needs officers. So the human immune system sends some of its cells to officer training schools in order to specialize. Their education begins at a tender age.

The bone marrow is the cradle of the immune system. From this protected nursery deep within you, brand new immune cells emerge every day. Some of these ultimately become the nonspecific cells that we discussed earlier, while others become lymphocytes. The latter are part of your specific immune system, so called because the cells can learn to recognize and recall specific targets. (Remember those lymphocytes sampling antigens on the macrophage's party tray.) That's why you become immune to something like chicken pox. Once these cells deal with an invading microorganism, they make a record of it, and they can zap it really fast the next time it shows up.

After the lymphocytes-to-be leave your bone marrow, some of them make their way to the thymus gland, a two-lobed organ at the top of your chest just under the base of your neck. After being "educated" in the thymus, they emerge as T-lymphocytes, or T-cells.

Another group of prelymphocytes stays in your bone marrow for continuing education and come out later as B-lymphocytes, or B-cells.

AGING: IT STARTS WITHIN

Time creaks on. And old age creeps up. As the biological clock ticks off the allotted span of a human life, the human body undergoes a series of age-related changes.

Athletic performance slows down. The 40-yard dash isn't as quick; the broad jump is not as broad; the ball doesn't fly as far. And what goes on inside the body reflects the more obvious changes on the outside. Some of the components of the immune system just don't pull together the way they used to.

"There are a number of functions we can measure that show reduced immune responsiveness in the elderly. Increasing chronological age correlates with immunodeficiency. The immune system never totally shuts off, it's just that its ability to respond is reduced," says Douglas Schmucker, Ph.D., professor of anatomy at the University of California in San Francisco and research scientist at the Veterans Administration Medical Center.

"This decline in immune function is probably an important reason for the increase in infectious diseases in the elderly. Nobody dies of 'old age.' People succumb to specific pathologies. Aging predisposes older people to pathologies such as pneumonia that young people would be able to respond to much more vigorously," explains Dr. Schmucker.

Researchers have found that aging shows up in two key areas of the immune system, according to Dr. Schmucker. The T-cells, important cells in fighting off infection, lose some of their ability to proliferate and to kill invaders. And since T-cells help the cells that make antibodies do their job, it's harder to get over an illness.

"Also, the incidence of autoimmunity goes up as we get older," says Dr. Schmucker. "Autoimmunity is the inability of the immune system to recognize self as self. The body will form antibodies against its own tissues and cells. Arthritis is one such autoimmune disease."

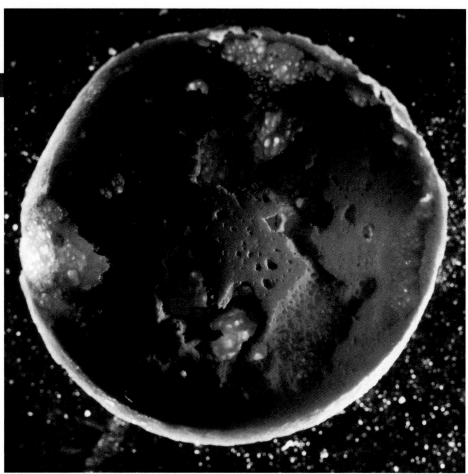

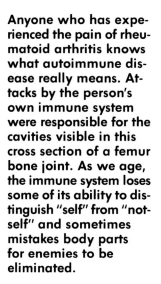
Anyone who has experienced the pain of rheumatoid arthritis knows what autoimmune disease really means. Attacks by the person's own immune system were responsible for the cavities visible in this cross section of a femur bone joint. As we age, the immune system loses some of its ability to distinguish "self" from "not-self" and sometimes mistakes body parts for enemies to be eliminated.

CHEMICAL SPEARS AND SWORDS

The millions of T-cells and B-cells go about their job of killing enemy invaders in a very different manner. One way of looking at it is that the B-cells throw spears from a distance while the T-cells engage in vicious cell-to-cell combat and stab the enemy with swords, explains the NIH's Dr. Lieber. The "spears" and "swords" are, of course, chemical in nature.

Each individual lymphocyte—depending on its unique chemical properties—is capable of reacting to only a small number of antigens. (Remember, an antigen is any microbe or substance that can stimulate an immune response.) That means that an antigen can be inside you and hundreds of lymphocytes can pass it and not recognize that it is an invader. *But,* and this is a big but, eventually the right lymphocyte will come in contact with the antigen and recognize it as a bad guy that has no business gallivanting about inside your body. When that particular lymphocyte goes into combat mode, the invader is in big trouble. There are millions of possible

antigens, but fortunately your immune system has lymphocytes capable of spotting every single one of them, explains Dr. Lieber.

Let's watch the B-cell in action. A B-cell doesn't move much. Let's say this particular B-cell is hanging around in one of your lymph nodes minding its own business. An antigen comes percolating through the lymph node. When the B-cell comes in contact with it, a message registers: *Wow. This stuff is dangerous. We'd better get into this fight.*

Like a caterpillar turning into a butterfly, the B-cell undergoes a marvelous transformation and turns into something called a plasma cell. The plasma cell starts pumping out antibodies specifically targeted for the antigen. The antibodies are like homing missiles, if you will, or spears that are tailor-made to stick on the particular enemy causing the trouble. If it's pneumonia bacteria involved in the invasion, the antibodies are specifically designed to glom on to pneumonia bacteria.

But one little plasma cell busy producing anti-

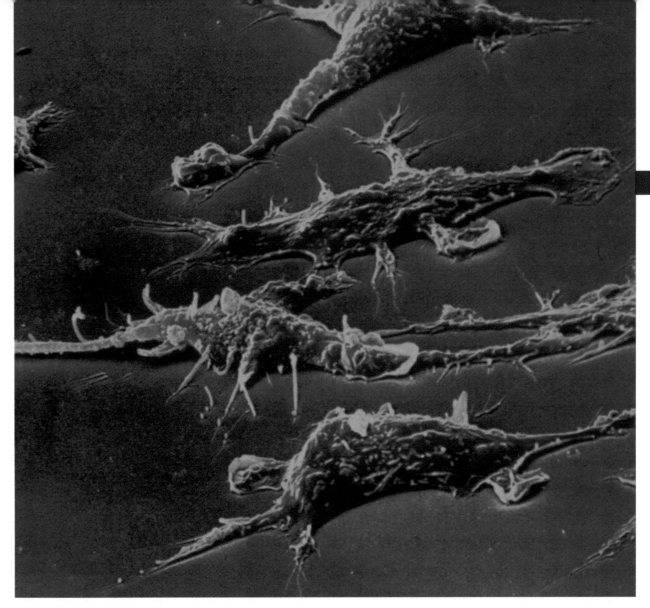

They look more like sci-fi blobs than something you can relate to personally, but macrophages are part of you. These relatively large (for cells, that is), slow-moving cells lie in wait for the chemical message that calls them to the scene of battle. Once they start eating bacteria, they liven up.

body missiles isn't going to push back a pneumonia infection. No problem. The plasma cell also starts dividing, producing exact copies of itself, which also start pumping antibodies. Soon there is a whole barrage of antibodies homing in on the invaders.

ANTIBODY AMMUNITION

Antibodies are tiny Y-shaped proteins with some pretty nifty properties, according to Dr. Lieber. After they leave the plasma cells and arrive at the battle scene, the forked section of their Y sticks onto the surface of the bacterium, or whatever. *Thoinggg*.

The other end of the Y, the pointy end, is like a chemical lock hanging out there looking for a chemical key that fits it. The chemical keys that do fit turn on some spectacular immunological fireworks. One of those keys is a type of protein produced by your body. This protein, known as complement, has nine components, and once one of them is attracted to the antibody, the other eight jump on as well. The antibodies and complement together explode the offending bacteria. Put the right key in the complement lock and KA-BAM! Goodbye, bacterium.

Antibodies and complement also make invaders much more palatable to macrophages and neutrophils. It's like putting a little savory sauce on the feast. If the antigen survives the chemical bomb provided by the antibodies and complement, the macrophages and neutrophils are still there to gobble it up.

Killer T-cells also make use of a lock and key

matchup. As the T-cells circulate throughout the body, their chemical keys hang out just looking for the chemical locks found on the surfaces of troublesome invaders.

MOPPING UP VIRUSES

T-cells are especially good at dealing with viruses and may have evolved for just that purpose, says Dr. Lieber. Viruses are particularly sneaky. Anywhere from 10 to 1,000 times *smaller* than bacteria, they take up residence *inside* your cells, thus escaping detection by neutrophils and macrophages.

If a virus that causes gastroenteritis, for example, makes its way through the membranes of your gastrointestinal tract, it looks for a home inside a cell. Without the help of your own DNA, it can't reproduce. But once inside your cell, it has just what it needs to raise a family.

It rapidly produces so many offspring that they literally burst the cell wall and spew out. Then each of these thousands of new viruses looks for its own home, yet another cell. Fortunately, when viruses slip inside your cells, they hang their coats outside. When the patrolling T-cell that has the particular chemical makeup to recognize that coat comes along, the intruder's game is up. It's like a husband coming home and finding a strange jacket in the hall closet. He *knows* what's going on upstairs in the bedroom.

The gastrointestinal tract cell with the virus inside and the telltale coat hanging on the outside is now viewed as an enemy. "It's kind of a defector. It's helping the virus procreate," says Dr. Lieber. "Just like in "Invasion of the Body Snatchers," the GI tract cell has been snatched. You could have compassion for it, because it's your own cell, but basically there's no hope for it. The T-cell has to kill that cell so that no more virus can be spewed out, so the T-cell goes up to the GI tract cell and pokes a hole in it."

Once a killer T-cell comes upon a cell that harbors a virus, it rapidly makes copies of itself so the copies can gang up on *all* the cells that have been invaded by viruses.

There are also T-cells known as helper cells. They tell the rest of the immune system how big a defense to mount, how many copies of B-cells or killer T-cells are needed. Other T-cells, known as suppressor cells, shut the defense off after the war is won. Not much is known about these types of cells, and their very existence is sometimes questioned, according to Dr. Lieber.

Once B-cells and T-cells have gone on the war-path against a particular antigen, a few cells or antibodies are kept in circulation just looking for the enemy to dare show its face again. That's where your acquired immunity to certain diseases comes from.

PSST, WHAT'S THE PASSWORD?

So how can the various components of the immune system tell an invader from, say, a red blood cell or a liver cell? Since immune cells don't have eyes with which to see the alien or ears with which to hear a whispered password, how do they know that the invaders are bad guys to be eliminated?

Every single cell in your body carries a pass card that identifies it as a part of you. This special arrangement of protein molecules says "self." Anything not so labeled is "not-self" and fair game for the immune system. As we age, though, the immune system loses some of its ability to make this distinction and sometimes attacks components of the body by mistake. When the immune system goofs and turns against the body, the results, known as autoimmune disease, can be devastating. (One such disease, in which the joints are attacked, is rheumatoid arthritis.)

But when things go right, as they usually do, your immune system loyally protects you from the surrounding horde of vicious viruses, malevolent microbes and bad-guy bacteria. The warfare it wages saves your life every day.

"Bacteria have no conscience. They just want to reproduce wherever they can," says Dr. Lieber. "Fortunately, your B-cells and T-cells have no conscience, either. They just do their job."

IMMUNITY AND CANCER

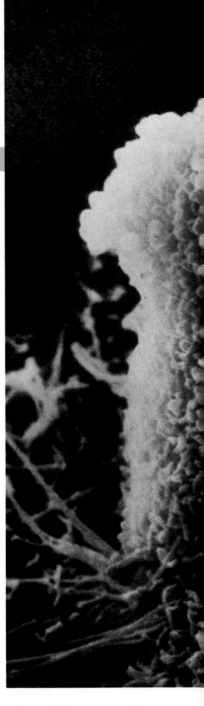

The party was perfect. Everyone had a good time. The steaks were grilled to a T. The before-dinner drinks, during-dinner drinks and after-dinner drinks kept the conversation alive. And that new air-freshening device—the one that automatically squirts perfume into the air every few minutes—kept anyone from noticing the cigarette smoke. Or the bug spray that nuked the mosquitoes.

But now you've got a problem. Because deep inside your body a wisp of smoke, a charred piece of meat or a dash of bug spray has turned on the grow light of a cell that could ultimately multiply out of control. And that means cancer.

"Cancer is something that goes on all the time in everybody," says Terry Phillips, Ph.D., associate professor of medicine and director of the Immunogenetics and Immunochemistry Laboratories at George Washington University Medical Center and coauthor of *Winning the War Within: Understanding, Protecting, and Building Your Body's Immunity.*

"Fortunately, the immune system copes with it 95 percent of the time—perhaps even 99 percent of the time. It's just that every so often your immune system is involved in something else or it shuts itself off."

Shuts itself *off?* Exactly. Sometimes it just gets exhausted by the load—cigarette smoke, sunlight, pesticides, viruses—that you hand it. So it turns itself off for a rest. And that's when you can get cancer.

The fluffy-looking little cell innocently tucked between these two "bullies" is actually an undercover cop for your immune system. It's checking their molecular I.D. When it's verified that the "bullies" are actually deadly cancer cells, the "cop" will reshape into a streamlined killer, punch a hole in each cancer cell and inject them with poison.

CALL THE POLICE

"The immune system is like the police force for your body," explains Dr. Phillips. It constantly patrols your streets checking the molecular I.D.'s of every cell. So when a cell changes—maybe a virus has moved in, for example—the officer examining that cell identifies the intruder and radios its I.D. to the nearest SWAT team. Then the sharpshooters surround the cell and shoot it down.

But what if there's a bacterial riot going on in your bladder at the same time? If your immune system's strong enough, says Dr. Phillips, it can fight on more than one front. And it will be if you learn

not to worry so much, get lots of sleep, exercise moderately, eliminate your contact with immune system depressants such as alcohol or tobacco, and eat a well-balanced diet. But what if you don't, and cancer gains a foothold?

MAGIC MESSENGERS

Fortunately, scientists can give your immune system a boost with magic messengers from their labs. They've figured out how to manufacture several components of your immune system that literally tell it how to fight the cancer.

Interferon, for example, is a chemical messen-

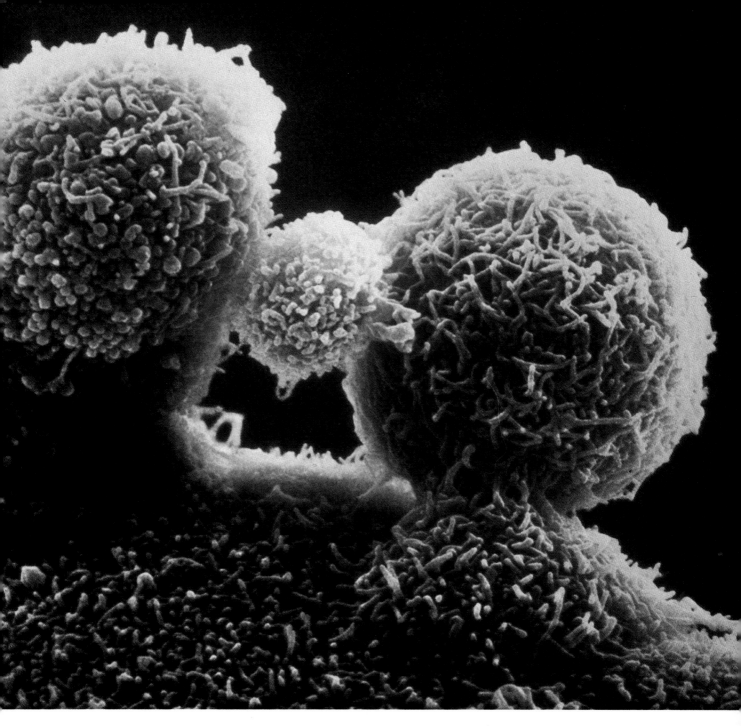

ger that the immune system uses as a frontline defense. It stimulates the "garbage-eating" cells—the macrophages—so that they are hyped for an attack whenever they get near a tumor.

For tumors that are inaccessible to macrophages, two other chemical messengers—interleukin 1 and 2—can be used to turbocharge your body's natural killer cells. "What we do," says Dr. Phillips, "is remove your tired lymphocytes and use the interleukin to give them new instructions that will fire them up. Then we put them back in your body."

Scientists can also make artificial antibodies—lobster-shaped warriors that grab cancer cells around the neck—then load them with cargos of toxic chemicals or lethal bacteria and target them at the cancer.

But the most effective weapon against cancer is—and probably always will be—early detection. "I think the biggest essential in cancer is that if you suspect something's wrong—you suddenly feel tired, you start to feel a little anemic—it's worth going to an internist," says Dr. Phillips. "And if there is any problem *whatsoever* that you don't feel comfortable about, ask for an opinion from an oncologist.

"If we catch cancer early enough and have a chance to boost the immune system," he says "we can get rid of it. Cancer *is* beatable."

INFECTION FIGHTING AT THE CDC

Not far from the Chattahoochee River, near a rambling road that smells of clay and pine, around the corner and down a ways from Dusty's Barbecue . . . someone is tabulating the incidence of leprosy in the United States in the past year. Or analyzing reports on toxic contamination levels of ceiling tiles in a public school in Madison, Wisconsin. Or showering in disinfectant after studying one of the deadliest diseases in the world.

The Centers for Disease Control (CDC), a federal agency headquartered in Atlanta, has played a leading role in the ongoing drama of modern medicine for more than 40 years. Among other accomplishments, the CDC took on the task of helping to eradicate from the world the scourge of smallpox; the last case was reported in 1977. And the CDC's aggressive immunization programs against infectious childhood diseases have made American children safer than ever from once-common infections like polio and whooping cough, measles and chicken pox.

Such ambitious programs haven't been without their problems, though. In 1976, the CDC's national campaign to immunize adults against swine flu virus resulted in uproar when some of the 50 million people who were vaccinated developed Guillain-Barré syndrome, a severe form of paralysis.

Whether in a national television program on controversial AIDS research or a newspaper story about a local outbreak of food poisoning, you've certainly heard about the CDC doing its taxpayer-supported duty to fight infection around the globe and in your own community.

DISEASE DETECTIVES

CDC employees report for work at an ever-expanding complex of nondescript concrete-and-steel buildings. It is in one such bland structure that the offices of the Epidemic Intelligence Service (EIS) sit near the end of a stark hallway, their rooms crammed with file cabinets and steel desks stacked high with paper. Nobody said it would be pretty. And nobody really seems to mind. This is, after all, home base for the CDC's rough and tough "disease detectives," a team of more than a hundred dedicated physicians, veterinarians, anthropologists, psychologists and public health laboratory scientists.

"Our job is to provide public service in times of public health emergencies," says Carl Tyler, M.D., director of the program. "We deal with everything from a food-borne infection that starts at a company picnic to what I regard as our most serious epidemic— the estimated 350,000 deaths a year that result from cigarette smoking."

Members of this elite epidemiology—or public health—program serve two-year stints in Atlanta or on assignment in various states. On call 24 hours a day, EIS officers are dispatched to investigate more than 3,000 health problems of epidemic proportion across the country every year.

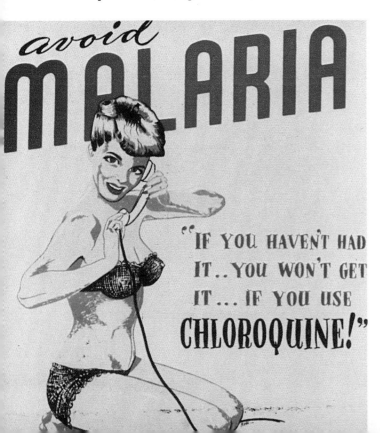

avoid MALARIA

"IF YOU HAVEN'T HAD IT . . YOU WON'T GET IT . . . IF YOU USE CHLOROQUINE!"

The CDC had its beginnings as the federal Office of Malaria Control in War Areas, established during World War II to control the disease in southern states. This 1942 pinup poster promoted use of an antimalaria medication.

Armed with questionnaires, lab equipment and seemingly boundless energy, EIS officers study mysterious new maladies daily. Take the case of the contaminated ice, for instance, when 158 football fans who attended a University of Pennsylvania-Cornell University game came down with viral gastroenteritis. Two days later, the same malady struck a crowd of 750 who attended a museum fund-raiser in Wilmington, Delaware. CDC's sleuths were able to link the outbreaks with beverages containing ice that was produced from well water that had been contaminated during a flood.

Since it may take several days before an epidemic becomes obvious, once the EIS is called, "We've got to get there fast, because we're reconstructing what happened, relying on people's memories," says Robert Gunn, M.D., assistant director of EIS officers assigned to state health departments. "It's somewhat like detective work. Let's say we suspect the food was contaminated. We ask everyone a series of well-designed questions. We ask the victims where they were, what they ate. We question the food handlers, ask them to reenact the steps they took in preparing things, try to determine if food was left out too long at inappropriate temperatures. We check out the kitchen, find delivery invoices and go to plants where the food came from.

"To do it right takes a lot of work. But it gives us lots of satisfaction to find the answers. And sometimes we come up with something really interesting."

The EIS pieced together the parts of the puzzle of Legionnaires' disease (see the accompanying box) and toxic shock syndrome (see the box "The Mystery That Was Toxic Shock" on page 24), and laboratory scientists at CDC were able to complete the picture. EIS officers who were conducting routine surveillance of various disease outbreaks in 1981 were the first to recognize what is now called AIDS.

More than 1,500 alumni have passed through the program. "We're building a top-flight team of world-class public health professionals," says Dr. Tyler. "A team we can call on any time, any place."

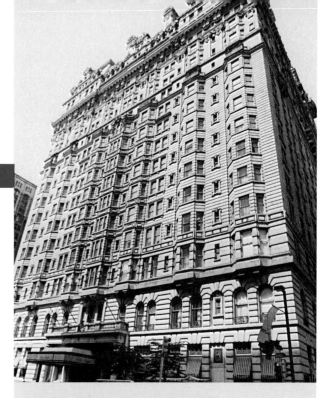

LEGIONS OF GERMS

In July 1976, a massive outbreak of acute respiratory illness—pneumonia in particular—struck a terrified turnout of tourists at the Bellevue-Stratford Hotel in Philadelphia. The unknown underlying illness was dubbed Legionnaires' disease, because most of the more than 200 victims—many of whom died—were attending an American Legion convention.

Reporting for immediate duty were some 30 officers of the Centers for Disease Control's Epidemic Intelligence Service, as well as laboratory scientists. Working long hours at a frantic pace, they raced from hospital to hospital interviewing victims, their families, friends and physicians. Floor by floor, they searched the hotel for the smallest clue. They pored over guest registries of other hotels and made hundreds of phone calls around the country to hunt for unreported victims who had already left town.

Finally, they began closing in: The disease, they determined, appeared to be transmitted through the air, not via person-to-person contact. Within six months, the CDC's team in Atlanta had pinned the culprit down: *Legionella pneumophila*—first in what would be an entire newly discovered strain of bacteria. Its hideout: the water in the Bellevue-Stratford's air-conditioning system.

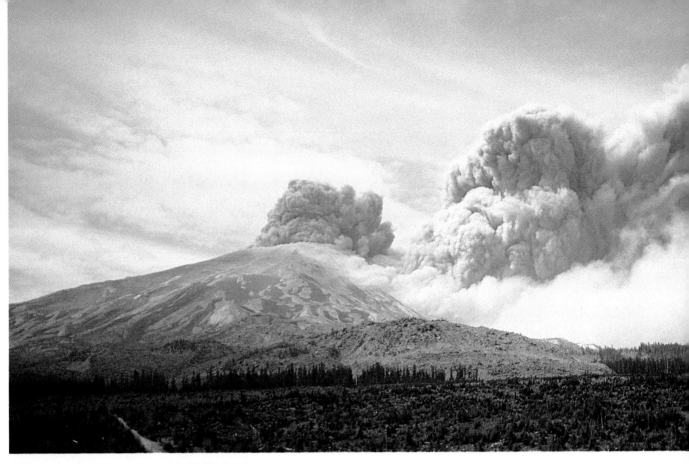

MEANWHILE, BACK AT THE LAB . . .

"Some people think that, thanks to vaccines, infectious diseases are all taken care of," says Ladine Newton, program manager of the CDC's Center for Infectious Diseases. "This isn't true. We don't know what new diseases we will be faced with next year."

Just how brimming with infection the world continues to be is reflected in the abundance of germs the CDC grapples with (specimens of which investigators send from the field to Atlanta for analysis). In fact, the CDC studies a wide diversity of diseases in microscopic detail on an everyday basis. There are the bacterial infections—such as pneumonia, tuberculosis and salmonellosis, or food poisoning; mycotic infections—those caused by fungi—such as histoplasmosis; parasitic diseases like malaria; and irritatingly persistent or frustratingly elusive viral diseases, which include everything from the common cold to influenza, from brain-swelling encephalitis to immunity-destroying AIDS.

More familiar diseases also receive the CDC's continued attention. "One of the most exciting areas," says Newton, "is identifying viruses that play a part in long-term health problems." CDC scientists are working with the human papilloma virus, which is linked to cervical cancer. They have also established a close tie between chronic viral hepatitis and the development of liver cancer.

"If there are new tools available, we use them. We get the best people and the latest technology into our laboratories," says Newton. "Our job is to control and prevent infectious diseases, whatever that takes."

DANGER: SCIENTISTS WORKING

The latest scientific technology is cramped for space in the CDC's "hot lab," research central for some of the deadliest diseases in the world.

"This laboratory is category P-4, requiring one of the highest levels of bio-containment," says Susan Fisher-Hoch, M.D., senior medical scientist of the special pathogens branch, division of viral diseases.

Dr. Fisher-Hoch's assistant meets visitors at a locked steel door. Inside, the dim hallway is punctuated with bright light emanating from glass-windowed labs, where men and women in white coats stare into microscopes and sit at long lab tables lined with glass test tubes and shimmering steel utensils. But these are mild, less invasive viruses they are working with, like hepatitis. The real killers are locked up deep behind more doors.

To enter the inner sanctum, Dr. Fisher-Hoch inserts a white plastic card with her personal code into the electronic security system slot beside the door. The door buzzes open.

"We study those diseases that are very dangerous,

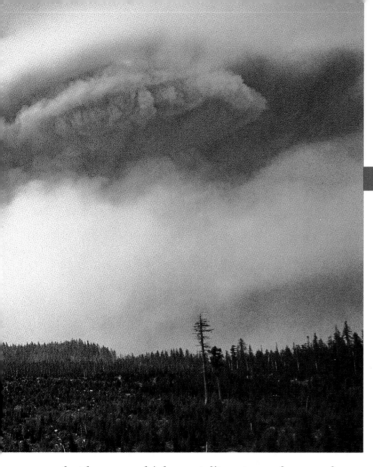

that have very high mortality rates and cause alarming outbreaks," she says. "Tropical diseases mostly."

Lassa fever, a potentially fatal disease that strikes thousands annually in West Africa, has been the object of Dr. Fisher-Hoch's scientific scrutiny for several years. In conjunction with the World Health Organization, the CDC has maintained a research project in Sierra Leone for more than a decade, which Dr. Fisher-Hoch visits as often as possible. Africa's Ebola-Marburg virus and the scourge of rural China, something called hemorrhagic fever with renal syndrome, are also high on the research priority list.

Studying some of the world's most lethal diseases while assuring that the researchers don't con-

tract them is a veritable study in antigerm warfare. Specimens of the deadly viruses are flown in to Atlanta from around the world, frozen solid in liquid nitrogen and immediately stored in freezer cases under tight security. The researchers don germproof suits before taking a single step in the direction of a deadly virus. And following a lab session, they shower—still in their suits—in disinfectant, then sterilize their equipment in a large, steam-jacketed tank to wipe out any surviving microbes.

The CDC's studies of tropical diseases, while certainly humanitarian, have a practical purpose. American travelers, workers and members of the armed forces in foreign countries are susceptible to exotic illnesses—as are the rest of us should the dangerous organisms responsible for them ever sneak across our borders undetected.

The researchers' years of work on Lassa fever are finally paying off: An effective antiviral drug treatment has been found, and they are testing a promising new vaccine in laboratory animals.

"Working here is very rewarding," says Dr. Fisher-Hoch. "We're accomplishing things in an area where nobody else is having any impact."

Germproof suits, completely enclosed and supplied with fresh air through hoses, protect "hot lab" researchers from contracting the deadly diseases they study.

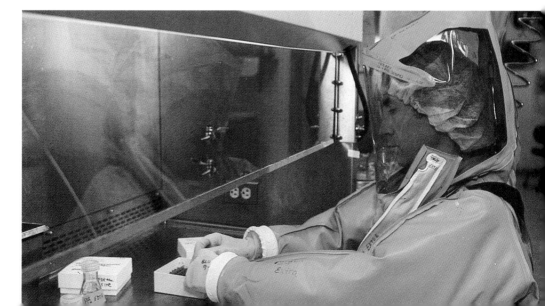

MEDICAL
FRONTIERS

The human immune system is at the epicenter of an explosion. The current star of the medical and scientific community, immunology research is mushrooming at a phenomenal rate. Knowledge doubles, then doubles again, piling up so quickly that researchers who have been in the field for years reel back in amazement.

"There are lots of interesting questions, and as you get answers, new questions become apparent, so it keeps moving forward," says John Fahey, M.D., director of the Center for Interdisciplinary Research in Immunology and Diseases at UCLA. "There's a lot of research still to do."

And all the while researchers will continually come up with mind-boggling strategies to boost human immunity. Here's a glimpse of what the future may hold for research and immunology.

CO-OPTING THE ENEMY

Viruses are insidious little creatures. They cause trouble out of all proportion to their size, slipping inside the cells of the human body with their nasty payload of disease and destruction.

Researchers are now working on ways to trick viruses into using their unsavory talents to ferry health rather than sickness into the body. The process, known as gene therapy, may someday provide a way to treat many serious illnesses caused by birth defects.

But before you can understand gene therapy, you have to understand what a virus is and how it works.

Viruses are like cellular vampires—they only stay alive by feeding on you, specifically your DNA, the genetic material within the nucleus of your cells. And just as when a vampire feeds on a victim, he also becomes a vampire, so some viruses—retroviruses —insert their own DNA into your genes so that whenever your cells reproduce, they make copies of the viruses' DNA as well.

INFECTED WITH HEALTH

Researchers have figured out how to harness the retroviruses' unique talents. They take snippets of DNA, genetic information that they *want* inserted into living cells, load it onto a retrovirus and let the virus carry it into the cell and insert it.

In a real sense, then, the gene therapy process coerces the virus into infecting the recipient with health rather than with a disease.

So far, gene therapy has been done only on experimental animals, but human trials are not far away, says leading researcher Inder Verma, Ph.D., professor of molecular biology at the Salk Institute in La Jolla, California.

"There is no scientific reason why it's not doable. It's like everybody knew you could go to the moon, but it was a long time before anybody went there. We're in the same place. We have all the tools," says Dr. Verma. "I would say, conservatively speaking, it's at least three to five years before someone attempts the human. On the other hand, science is moving so fast it could be closer than that."

And when someone does attempt to use viruses to ferry this microscopic payload into human cells, what kind of genetic information would scientists like inserted?

Dr. Verma predicts that the first trials will be on children suffering from SCID. That is Severe Combined Immunodeficiency Disease, the birth defect that kept the famous Bubble Boy locked into a sterile environment because he didn't have a functioning immune system. Other diseases that researchers might attempt to correct early on would be thalassemia, a type of anemia necessitating lifelong blood transfusions, and hemophilia, a lifethreatening disease in which the blood fails to clot.

Ready for a close-up look at the stuff of life? Using the technology of 3-D crystallography, a method that uses X-rays to take photographs of very small objects, scientists can create models of the very molecules that make up your body. This is a computer model of a strand of DNA. Focusing in on the molecular structures of viruses and DNA helps scientists design new drugs to augment your immune system's disease-fighting ability.

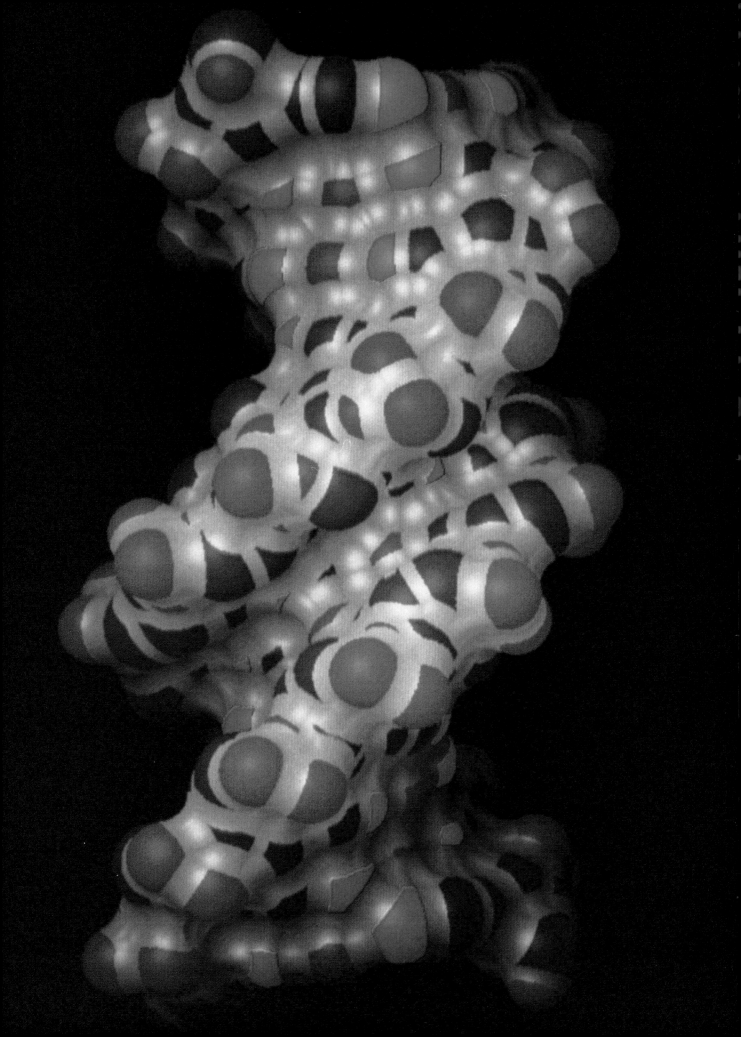

These birth defects are better understood in terms of genetics than some other diseases that involve more complex biological processes. But someday, someday in the more distant future, doctors may be able to use gene therapy to correct diseases like cystic fibrosis, diabetes and some types of muscular dystrophy, says Dr. Verma. Someday genetic defects that underlie these diseases may even be corrected while the fetus is still in the womb.

Dr. Verma is not surprised that science is harnessing viruses. "Take the case of the fungi," he says. "For years and years fungi caused disease, yet it is the fungi that give us antibiotics—penicillin, streptomycin, tetracycline. So in a way it's not surprising that we should use the retroviruses. I guess the surprise is the human ingenuity to use something that is potentially dangerous and turn it into a very useful thing."

SUBJUGATING THE CANCER MONSTER

Viruses can be tricked. But what about cancer? Cancer presents such a major challenge to the immune system that sometimes the body just gives up. Now even cancer seems to be yielding before the onslaught of immunology research.

In some laboratories around the country, scientists are tricking tumor cells into making medicines that show promise as new weapons against cancer and other dread diseases. Tumor cells from mice, specifically B-cells from their immune systems, are being combined with human cells and stimulated to produce a whole host of new protective antibodies.

Such mouse/man products are known as "monoclonal antibodies" or "engineered antibodies," says Terry Phillips, Ph.D., associate professor of medicine and director of the Immunogenetics and Immunochemistry Laboratories at George Washington University Medical Center and coauthor of *Winning the War Within: Understanding, Protecting, and Building Your Body's Immunity.*

Dr. Phillips's particular area of interest is "idio-

type" and "anti-idiotype" antibodies. Antibodies are complex proteins that your immune system produces to fight specific diseases. (For a more detailed explanation, see the entry on how your immune system works, beginning on page 50.) It seems that when the B-cells of your immune system produce antibodies against a disease, they also produce a whole cascade of related antibodies that can enhance or shut down the fight against that particular disease. These are the "idiotypes" and "anti-idiotypes."

When the immune system of a person who has cancer gives up, it's a sign that the idiotypic antibody has moved in. Depending upon the stress levels and nutritional levels of the patient, the immune system sometimes just raises a white flag and stops fighting, says Dr. Phillips. Researchers are hoping to harvest from cancer patients the anti-idiotypic antibody produced in the early stages of their cancer, the antibody that can switch the immune response back on.

"We could take the antibodies from patients in the early stages, store the cells, resurrect them, and make human monoclonal antibodies for treatment regimens later on when they start to lose control of the tumor," says Dr. Phillips.

CREATING NEW WEAPONS

If these idiotypic antibodies work the way researchers think they're going to work, a whole host of new vaccines may be possible, according to Dr. Phillips. Vaccines that switch off the immune system when it's too zealous could put the dampers on autoimmune diseases such as diabetes or rheumatoid arthritis. Allergic responses may be tamed. Organ transplants, currently plagued by the immune system's attempts to reject the transplanted tissues, would be safer.

The components of this line of engineered vaccines would be made from cells taken from the individual receiving the vaccine. Some researchers are now using human tumor cells, rather than mouse cells, to conduct their research. That makes the end product *almost* you. All this research may someday lead to a line of drugs custom designed just for you.

"You would be using your own material and

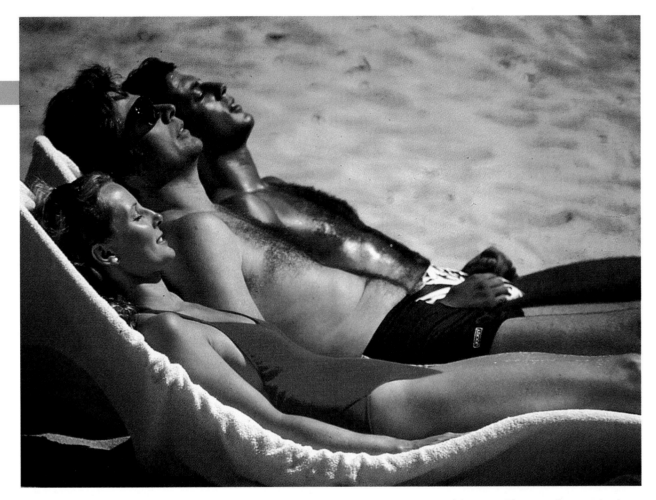

therefore we wouldn't be introducing extraneous drugs into the system," says Dr. Phillips. "We'd actually be introducing almost your own individual generic drug, which is the exciting thing about this. We'd use you to engineer your own therapy. I'm looking to the time we wouldn't even have to engineer this stuff. You would be able to come in to a specialized clinic and donate blood. The blood would be grown and stimulated and the antibodies would be harvested from your own material, purified and given back."

If that's not enough to make viruses and bacteria shake in their boots, other researchers are taking different paths in the endless quest for new weapons against disease.

MEDICAL ENGINEERING

New drugs used to be "mixed" or "discovered" or even "invented."

Suddenly, new drugs are being "engineered." Researchers are studying on a molecular level the shapes of viruses and the way they function. And

Attention sun worshippers. The good news is that at last medical researchers have succeeded in creating a vaccine against melanoma, the most dangerous—and often fatal—type of skin cancer. Sun damage is considered to be a prime cause of the dread disease. The bad news is that the vaccine is being used only on people who already have the disease. But even if the day comes when it becomes available to the general public, it would not replace the best preventive that doctors have been pitching for years: Wear sunscreen and limit your exposure to the sun's rays.

they are shaping drugs whose molecules plug into viral molecular structures. It sounds complicated, but basically it's a strategy to gum up the working parts in a virus.

Viruses have so far escaped the best efforts of medical science. Bacteria succumb to antibiotics, but such medications don't touch viruses. There just isn't much in the way of readily available drugs to go after these troublesome microbes.

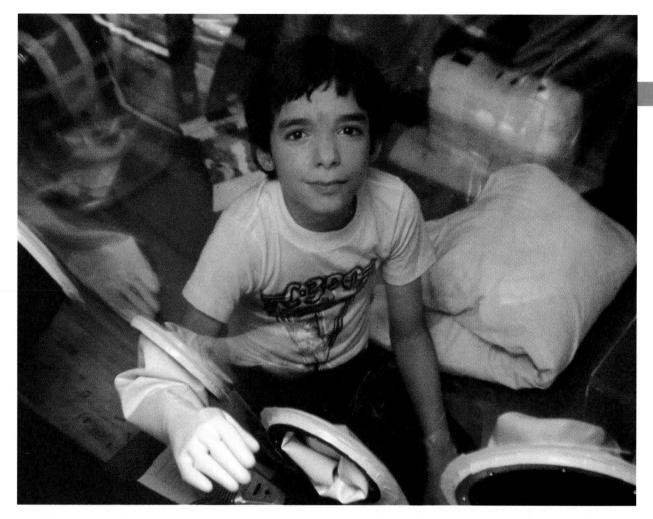

Viruses are small. The polio virus, for example, is so small that if you imagined an *E. coli* bacterium (*E. coli* bacteria live in your intestines and help you digest your food) to be the size of a football field, the polio virus would be about the size of the football.

They are not too small to escape scientific scrutiny, however. Researchers are using a process known as 3-D crystallography to get a closer look at how viruses work, according to John McGowan, Ph.D., chief of the Developmental Therapeutics Branch AIDS Program, at the National Institute of Allergy and Infectious Diseases.

The 3-D crystallography method works by putting crystallized material—and viruses form very nice crystals—onto a platform and bombarding it with X-rays. The reflections are caught on film and the image enhanced by computer.

The process has been around for a number of years, but its use with viruses is only now revealing how viruses function and may lead to the develop-

For a child born without a functioning immune system, the world is a hostile place. David, who was born in 1971 with SCID (Severe Combined Immunodeficiency Disease), spent his short life in a totally germ-free environment. He became famous as the Bubble Boy. Researchers think the day is approaching when a revolutionary technique known as gene therapy will enable babies born with SCID to lead normal lives.

ment of new drugs to block them.

Viruses are proteins, and proteins "don't exist as rigid structures," explains Dr. McGowan. "If you held out your hand and opened and closed it, that's the concept of what proteins do to interact with other proteins inside your body."

Once scientists understand the way that viruses need to move in order to invade the cells of the human body, they can design a drug that fools the virus, says Dr. McGowan.

"Understanding structures is a new key way for

developing new drugs. You're mimicking what the virus normally grabs onto so it thinks it's grabbing onto that. You're tricking it so it can't let go and, in effect, you've stopped it."

In the future, such structures engineered to fit into viruses may hold some hope for AIDS sufferers, says Dr. McGowan.

MOVING BEYOND DRUGS

While some scientists wrestle over exotic new drugs and sophisticated bio-tech methodology, others are getting really basic. They're looking at the connections between diet and the immune system.

Does what you eat, or don't eat, influence whether you resist infection? Does your diet have any impact on how fast you heal?

Long-term restriction of your caloric intake may make your immune system hold up better as you age, believes Richard Weindruch, Ph.D., health scientist administrator at the National Institute on Aging and coauthor with UCLA's Roy Walford, M.D., of *The Retardation of Aging and Disease by Dietary Restriction.* Work with experimental animals has shown that the immune system ages at a slower rate in animals fed a highly nutritious but reduced-calorie diet for long periods.

"Most of the immune functions that change with age stay younger longer in the animals that had this restricted diet. The ability of T-lymphocytes [important defense cells of the immune system] to proliferate goes down with age and goes up with long-term dietary restriction. The ability of T-cells to kill tumor cells goes down with advancing age and stays higher with dietary restriction," explains Dr. Weindruch.

"The immune system is one of several systems that go awry with aging, and it's obvious that it would produce health benefits if the immune system were kept intact as the organism ages," he says.

The dietary research on experimental animals may alter medical recommendations for human diet in the future, Dr. Weindruch predicts. "Twenty or 30 years ago, the goal of nutrition was to promote rapid growth. That was the standard. The quicker you grew, the better the diet. This research has shown quite clearly that diets that seek explosive growth are not those that are associated with long life and late onset of disease."

The day may come, he says, in which parents worry that their children are growing too rapidly. Gone would be the anxious parent forcing children to eat more so they'll grow up big and strong. And adults might nibble salads, not out of concern for their waistlines, but in hopes that their immune systems will help keep them younger longer.

MIND GAMES

Researchers in the new field of psychoneuroimmunology are learning more every day about how mental attitudes affect the immune system. They've found that negative emotions—stress, depression, grief—suppress some immune functions. Some researchers are now trying to figure out ways to use the mind to *enhance* immune function.

Someday a person might sniff an aroma or listen to a particular song as part of cancer treatment, say scientific researchers at the University of Alabama in Birmingham. They are conditioning the immune systems of experimental animals. The animals smell the penetrating odor of camphor before being injected with a drug that revs up some functions of their immune systems. After several trials, the animals' immune systems respond when the animal merely sniffs the odor and does not receive the drug.

If a particular song were paired with the aroma, the researchers believe, it might be possible to give less drug by just having the patient listen to the song.

Fine, you say, but when are they going to come up with a cure for the common cold?

Hang in there. Richard Colonno, Ph.D., director of anti-viral research at Merck Sharp & Dohme Division, Merck & Company in West Point, Pennsylvania, is working on engineering a drug that should fit into the structure of most cold viruses and prevent them from infecting you.

MEDICATIONS

For most of us, catching any sort of infectious disease can be a test of our patience. But only two or three generations ago, getting sick was a test of survival. In our great-grandmother's day, infections spread fast through entire populations, often with fatal results.

When we get sick today, we generally suffer fewer symptoms and get well a lot faster than our forebears did—and rarely do we fear for our lives. What accounts for this profound change? Antibiotics— the amazing medications that work together with our immune systems to battle against infection.

"Antibiotics have opened up the 'golden age' of medicine," says Alvin B. Segelman, Ph.D., associate professor of pharmacognosy at Rutgers University and coauthor of *Antibiotics in Historical Perspective*.

It all started with the serendipitous—some would say downright sloppy—discovery of the first antibiotic,

penicillin, by Alexander Fleming in 1928. A scientist who had the habit of keeping dishes of bacteria cultures sitting out for long periods on his laboratory workbench, Fleming one day noticed that a bit of mold growing on a culture was killing the bacteria. He isolated the mold's powerful antibacterial factor and named it penicillin, and it was successfully tested on hospital patients. The rest, as they say, is history. Thousands of types of penicillin and other antibiotics have been discovered or synthesized in laboratories since then, says Dr. Segelman, and scientists are developing new ones every day.

Antibiotics belong to a group of medications that wage war on microbes—the microscopic organisms that can produce infection in human beings. These antimicrobials include drugs that combat bacteria and similar organisms (like those that cause syphilis and Rocky Mountain spotted fever).

DRUGS FOR AN IMMUNE SYSTEM GONE AMOK

What could be more marvelous than the human immune system? An immune system that doesn't make mistakes. Errors of judgment by this powerful regulator of health can result in serious disorders called autoimmune diseases. Rheumatoid arthritis, inflammatory bowel disease and multiple sclerosis are a few examples. The problem, scientists believe, is that some people's immune systems mistakenly identify normal cells as foreign invaders. When that happens, a destructive attack is mounted against the person's own innocent tissues.

Thanks to medications known as immuno-suppressants, however, faulty immune systems can be slowed down in their misguided advances. Some of these drugs do their job by searching for rapidly dividing immune cells and then killing them before they can do their damage, explains Michael Lieber, M.D., Ph.D., an immunologist at the National Institutes of Health.

These antiproliferation drugs are generally prescribed for severe autoimmune diseases.

Corticosteroids, another form of immunosuppressant (different from muscle-building anabolic steroids), are crucial for the survival of people who have received organ transplants. Without such drugs, their immune systems would automatically reject tissues foreign to the body—and another person's liver or heart is about as foreign as can be. Transplant patients taking this drug—which they must do for a lifetime—are more suspectible to every type of infection, however. Cyclosporine, a relatively new drug for organ recipients, poses less of a problem.

Antihistamines are a type of immunosuppressant drug familiar to most people with allergies or hay fever. They prevent the inflammation-causing effects of a body chemical called histamine.

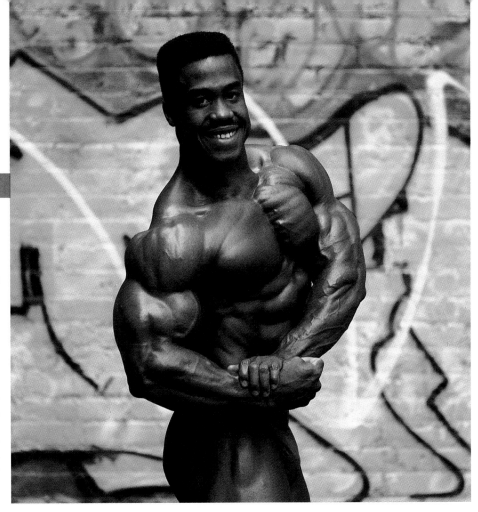

Nationally ranked body-builder Mike Ashley takes a tough stance against anabolic steroids, which some athletes use to increase muscle and boost athletic performance. Physicians who advise bodybuilders warn that habitually taking these drugs — a form of the male hormone testosterone — may compromise the immune system and lead to cancer, liver damage and other serious problems.

By far, penicillin is the biggest kid on the infection-fighting block. The most commonly prescribed antibiotic in the world, it's used to treat everything from respiratory infections to gonorrhea. About one person in ten is allergic to the drug, however, and may experience swelling, breathing difficulties, severe itching, hives and—in rare cases—death. You probably won't discover you're allergic, unfortunately, until you have a reaction. But if you are, your doctor has plenty of alternatives. *Tetracyclines* are frequently substituted and are particularly useful against respiratory infections.

Cephalosporins are another popular type of antibiotic. Then there are aminoglycosides, such as streptomycin, which are used for serious infections like tuberculosis. Macrolides, such as erythromycin, are commonly prescribed to treat children's ear, throat and skin infections. Sulfa drugs are often effective against urinary tract infections. Polymyxins and chloramphenicol are used for especially serious infections.

Your doctor's choice of an appropriate medication for your infection depends upon several factors. Most obviously, some drugs are more effective than others in treating certain diseases, and you also

need to steer clear of any drugs you're allergic to. Your doctor may also have professional preferences for specific drugs. And in some cases you may be given a brand-new medication you've never heard of before; new drugs are constantly being developed to replace old ones that disease-causing microbes have become cunningly resistant to.

Whatever medication your doctor prescribes, be sure to follow the instructions carefully, says Dr. Segelman. Even if you feel better before your prescription runs out, keep taking your medicine to assure that the infection is completely wiped out.

And don't ever share someone else's prescription, he cautions. "It's very dangerous. You may be taking the wrong medication—an antibiotic is totally ineffective against a virus, for instance—and your infection will just get worse."

Antibiotics certainly qualify as miracle workers, but the real miracle is your body's ability to use them to heal itself. People on powerful medications may still not survive disease if their immune systems aren't strong. So don't count on medicine alone to come to your rescue. Instead, do your best to keep your immune system in tip-top shape—and you may rarely need medications in the first place.

MEDICATIONS THAT HELP THE IMMUNE SYSTEM

Your immune system benefits from medication in numerous ways. Some simply slow microbes down while your system produces infection-fighting antibodies. Others directly stimulate the production of immune cells. The medications described here comprise the major types prescribed by physicians. For complete information on these and other medications, consult your doctor or refer to printed materials that accompany your prescriptions.

TYPE OF MEDICATION	ACTION AND APPLICATION	CAUTIONS AND SIDE EFFECTS
Antimicrobials		
Penicillins	Help the immune system by weakening certain types of bacteria. Used in treating streptococcal, pneumococcal and staphyloccocal infections; gonorrhea; syphilis and meningococcal meningitis.	Allergic reactions may occur. Prolonged use may cause skin rashes and overgrowth of nonsusceptible organisms such as fungi.
Cephalosporins Semisynthetic antibiotics, such as Beta-Lactim, with actions similar to penicillin.	Beta-Lactim used to treat urinogenital infections. Other types effective against minor infections from many varieties of bacteria.	Reactions may be similar to those of penicillin. Do not use if you are allergic to penicillin. May not be safe for use by pregnant women.
Macrolides Antibiotics such as erythromycin.	Useful in treating upper respiratory tract infections and urethral infections caused by chlamydia. Also active against parasitic amoeba and syphilis.	Allergic reactions can occur. Can cause liver failure in patients with impaired liver function. Also can cause gastrointestinal upsets and abdominal cramps. Do not use if taking theophyllin.
Lincosamides Very powerful antibiotics such as lincomycin and clindamycin.	Effective in combating staphylococcal infections that are resistant to less powerful antibiotics. Used in treating syphilis.	Allergic reactions can occur. May cause gastrointestinal upsets, skin rashes, vertigo, vaginitis and loss of blood platelets. Do not take for minor infections. Extra care should be taken if you are taking drugs for high blood pressure.
Tetracyclines	Effective against a wide range of bacteria, especially those that cause conjunctivitis, acne and urethral, vaginal and rectal infections.	Allergic reactions can occur as well as skin rashes, anemia, nausea, vomiting and infections in the vagina and rectum. Women who are breastfeeding should not take these drugs, as they may harm an infant's developing teeth and bones.
Chloramphenicol A powerful drug reserved for serious infections.	Used to combat such heavy hitters as typhus, typhoid, cholera and hemolytic influenza.	Among other side effects are headaches, mental confusion and delirium, gastrointestinal upsets and serious blood disorders.
Trimethoprim	Used to treat urinary tract infections due to *E. coli*, Klebsiella and staphylococci bacteria.	Can cause allergic reactions, skin rashes, nausea, vomiting, anemia and fever. Do not use while taking phenytoin.
Sulfonamides	Sulfa-containing drugs weaken bacteria. Effective in treating acute urinary tract infections, pyelonephritis, cystitis, otitis media and Chloriquine-resistant malaria.	Among other side effects are anemia, skin rashes, hepatitis, convulsions, depression and insomnia. Do not use with diuretics. May be hazardous for pregnant and nursing mothers.
Topical Anti-Infective Agents (also called antiseptics)	These creams and ointments, used to cover cuts, burns and other injuries to the skin, weaken or kill skin bacteria. This aids the immune system's macrophages in their task of keeping the skin clean.	Often cause localized skin reactions and secondary bacterial infections. Many mixtures contain cortisol, which suppresses action of the skin macrophages. Do not use along with antihistamines or corticosteroid-containing creams.

TYPE OF MEDICATION	ACTION AND APPLICATION	CAUTIONS AND SIDE EFFECTS
Antimycobacterial Agents	Help the immune system combat tuberculosis by inhibiting the growth of the tubercle bacillus.	Can cause headache, fatigue, mental confusion, muscle weakness, allergic and renal complications and possibly anemia and loss of blood platelets. Do not use with other drugs.
Antiparasitics		
Antifungal Agents	Effective in controlling fungal infections such as ringworm by competing with the fungus for food. Very helpful because the immune system cannot readily overcome fungal infections.	Can produce allergic reactions. Do not use with oral contraceptives, barbiturates or anticoagulation therapy.
Antiprotozoal Agents	These drugs kill protozoa by poisoning them or by inhibiting their ability to take in food. Effective in treating turista, diarrhea and malaria.	Can produce liver and renal complications and other symptoms associated with heavy metal poisoning.
Antihelmintics	Kill parasitic worms like tapeworms and roundworms by poisoning them or inhibiting their ability to take in food.	Can produce liver and renal complications and other symptoms associated with heavy metal poisoning.
Antiviral Agents		
Acyclovir	Retards the growth of viruses such as herpes by inhibiting their ability to infect cells. Also helps the immune system recognize infected cells.	Adverse reactions vary widely. Consult the guidelines accompanying your particular medication.
Immune-Modulating Agents		
Interferons	The alpha and beta are naturally produced by the body to help combat viruses until specific antibodies are produced. Gamma interferon is made by the lymphocytes and is an activator of macrophages. Used in dressing wounds. Also somewhat useful against cancer.	Adverse effects are not known.
Interleukin	These molecular communicators stimulate activation and proliferation of immune system cells. They are used experimentally to treat cancer and immune deficiencies.	Adverse effects are not known.
Immune Globulin	These are antibodies present in human serum. Given to people lacking in natural antibody protection, they provide overall protection against a wide variety of bacteria and viruses.	Can produce serum sickness and kidney complications. Because they are given intravenously, they present the risk of AIDS and other diseases transmitted via blood transfusions.
Inosiplex	This experimental drug is both an antiviral agent and a stimulant to the immune system. It stimulates immune system T-cells into action against virus-infected cells.	Excessive use can lead to overstimulation of the immune system and promotion of the growth of the other viruses and bacteria. Do not take with other immune system stimulants.

YOUR MIND AND YOUR IMMUNE SYSTEM

A man dying of cancer gets an injection of distilled water that he believes to be a brand-new superdrug. His tumors disappear. When he later reads in the newspaper that the new treatment has proved worthless, his cancer comes back and he dies.

A 16-year-old boy is shunned by friends and teachers because he is suffering from a disfiguring skin disease, congenital ichthyosiform erythroderma. The condition, characterized by dark, fishlike scales on the body, is thought to be incurable. But when the boy is hypnotized, the hardened scales drop away in a few days, revealing fresh, normal-looking skin.

A woman who suffers severe allergic reactions to roses is sitting in her doctor's office. The doctor takes an exquisite rose from behind a screen and holds it in his hand. When she sees it, she suffers a full-blown allergic attack. The rose is artificial.

What's going on here? Can it be that your thoughts can make you sick? Can your thoughts also heal you?

For most of the 20th century, microbes held center stage. If you asked a physician what caused disease, the answer would come, sure and simple. Germs. Viruses. Bacteria. Parasites. Tiny little creatures that invade the body and do their dirty work.

Not that doctors were unaware that the mind somehow played a role in disease and healing. After all, healers have known about and made use of the power of suggestion (the placebo effect) for thousands of years. It's just that thoughts can't be put in a test tube and measured. Emotions can't be viewed under a microscope. The modern mechanistic view of "one disease, one microbe, one cure" was so tidy. It put things in a neat little package. The problem is, the package just won't float anymore.

THE MIND'S ROLE MATTERS

Recent research into the connection between the mind and the immune system has opened a door that promises to revolutionize medicine. Germs are no longer the only villains of the show. They aren't about to do a disappearing act, but they are going to have to move over and share the stage with such factors as stress, grief, anxiety and depression.

"The immune system is not some mindless automaton that runs parallel to our conscious experience of the world but detached from it. The immune system is in constant communication or dialogue with the brain. And the brain and nervous system are in constant dialogue and communication with the immune system," says David Sobel, M.D., coauthor of *The Healing Brain.*

The "conversation" between the brain and the immune system is a highly complicated affair. Scientists are just beginning to eavesdrop on that conversation. The whisperings that they've heard so far open up a new world for medical exploration—the field of psychoneuroimmunology. It is a science that looks at health and disease in terms of the nervous system, the immune system and the mind.

EMOTIONS THAT PROTECT

"I think it's going to lead to a whole new way of thinking about health and illness," says George Solomon, M.D., professor of psychiatry at UCLA and one of the first Americans to study the connections between psychological states and immunity.

Dr. Solomon's early work with psychologist Rudolph H. Moos, Ph.D., focused on rheumatoid arthritis patients and their families. Rheumatoid arthritis is an autoimmune disease in which an individual's immune system somehow produces antibodies that attack the body's defenses, showing up in the blood as rheumatoid factor. Joint pain and inflammation result.

Dr. Solomon and Dr. Moos's study found that some relatives of people with this disease had rheumatoid factor in their blood also, but were not suffering any debilitating effects. The people who had the blood factor but not the inflammation and pain shared one unique feature—compared to the general population they scored high on tests rating their emotional health.

"We felt that their good emotional health protected them from rheumatoid arthritis," says Dr.

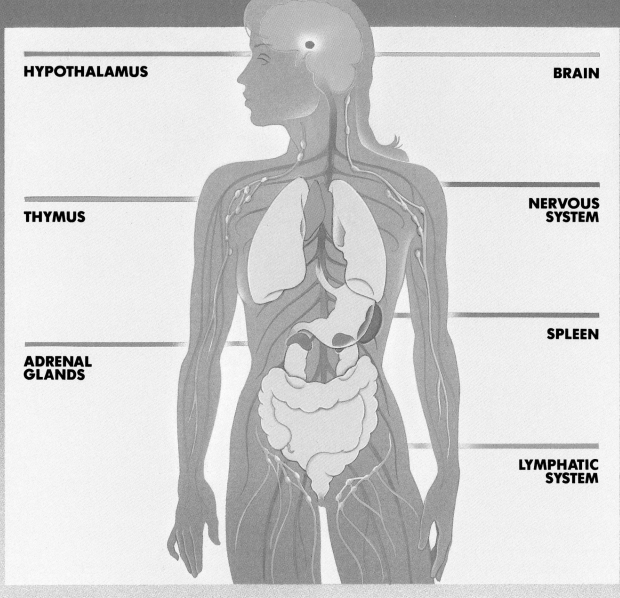

HYPOTHALAMUS

THYMUS

ADRENAL
GLANDS

BRAIN

NERVOUS
SYSTEM

SPLEEN

LYMPHATIC
SYSTEM

THE BRAIN/BODY CONNECTION

They are cells, hundreds of times tinier than the period at the end of this sentence. But when you feel bad, they feel it, too. Scientists say that grief, for example, literally kills one type of protective immune cell. Other immune cells may become more sluggish than normal.

The full communications system between mind and body has not yet been mapped out, but scientists have uncovered a number of ways through which your emotions may reach out and touch your immune system.

A network of nerves supplies a direct connection between the brain and a number of organs important to your immune system—the thymus, spleen and lymph nodes. Immune cells from your bone marrow and thymus travel through the

lymphatic system to lymph nodes and spleen, where they serve as a sort of reserve of combat cells ready to go into action should the need arise.

In addition to direct nerve connections, there is also a variety of chemicals used for communication. The hypothalamus, a portion of the brain, manufactures hormones that in turn cause the release of adrenal hormones—epinephrine, norepinephrine and corticosteroids. They in turn can affect the immune system.

There are receptors on some immune cells for neurotransmitters, chemicals that the brain uses to communicate. The communication may very well be two-way. Some immune cells manufacture beta-endorphins and other chemicals that may help control mood in the brain.

Is it a butterfly? A bird? Would you believe a predictor of cancer? A study at Johns Hopkins University School of Medicine followed for a number of years students who took a Rorschach test (a portrayer of psychological health). Those who revealed unsatisfactory interpersonal relationships proved more likely to develop cancer later in life.

Solomon. If any of these people were to become depressed or unable to deal with severe stress, they would be well advised to seek counseling immediately, because "they would probably be at risk of developing the disease."

Even now, similar studies are under way to determine why some people who have been exposed to the AIDS virus and who have antibodies to the virus in their blood for several years have not come down with the disease, says Dr. Solomon. Could it be, he asks, that their emotional health, acting through brain/immune system connections, is protecting them—at least for a while?

And what about cancer, another illness that features an immune system gone awry? The existence of a so-called cancer personality is still controversial, but doctors have noted that some cancer patients tend to fit the "nice guy" mold, passive patients who don't complain. One researcher found that the patients with the fastest-growing tumors were often "consistently serious, overcooperative, overnice, overanxious, painfully sensitive, passive,

apologetic personalities." But the fighters, those who are angry and determined to beat the dread disease, tend to survive longer.

Dr. Solomon maintains that in *all* disease, a multitude of factors—including the emotional—is at work in both the onset of the illness and how it runs its course.

GRIEF ZAPS IMMUNITY

Since Dr. Solomon's pioneering work on arthritis, other scientists have found evidence that negative emotions have an impact on the immune system.

Helplessness, hopelessness, depression, grief and despair seem to be the most destructive emotions in terms of immunity, says Dr. Solomon.

Take grief, for example. Grief hurts, apparently right down to the cellular level.

Everyone has heard the stories of loving couples following each other to the grave: Uncle Charlie doted on Aunt May for decades. He cared for her when she was infirm and hovered solicitously over her hospital bed as she lay dying. Although Uncle

Charlie seemed in the best of health, two months after Aunt May died, he came down with pneumonia. And he died.

Once people would have said Uncle Charlie died of a broken heart. What he *really* died of may have been an impaired immune system.

A number of studies have looked into the biology of people suffering bereavement and found that their immune systems also suffer.

One Australian study followed the lives of 26 people whose spouses had died from either accident or illness. In addition to offering counseling services to the bereaved, researchers took blood samples. They found that the immune systems of the bereaved were temporarily weakened. The T-cells, a type of immune cell that attacks invading microorganisms, were slower to react.

A more recent California study examined the blood of women whose husbands had just died. Their natural killer cells, another important component of the immune system, showed reduced activity.

DISCORD, THEN DISEASE?

Like bereavement, separation and divorce also leave their mark on the immune system.

A couple gets into an argument about money or sloppy housekeeping or whatever else married couples argue about. They get into another argument and yet another. Finally, they separate. Because they raise their voices, the whole neighborhood follows the deterioration of their marriage. The whole neighborhood listens in. But the neighbors may not be the only ones eavesdropping.

It seems the very cells of their immune systems, the cells whose job it is to patrol the body and keep out invading viruses, may be listening as well. They may "hear" the commotion and somehow feel the stress and depression. And, more important, they may slow down on the job as a result.

Studies at Ohio State University certainly point in that direction. Janice Kiecolt-Glaser, Ph.D., Ronald Glaser, Ph.D., and their colleagues at Ohio State University studied the immune systems of women

TYPE A'S AND CANCER

A is for Type A, the hard-driven, stressed-out personality. B is for the more relaxed personality. C is for cancer. The ABC's of cancer, spelled out in one study, are that Type A's face a greater risk of dying of cancer than Type B's.

In 1960 and 1961, researchers at Boston University School of Medicine classified over 3,000 men into the two categories. By 1983, 186 men had died of cancer—112 Type A's and 74 Type B's.

After accounting for age and lifestyle, the researchers concluded that the incidence of death in Type A's from cancers other than lung cancer was more than 1½ times that of the Type B's.

A possible explanation: Type A's see life as a series of challenges and are frustrated when things go wrong. Their frustrations over losing control may impair their immune systems, making them more susceptible to cancer.

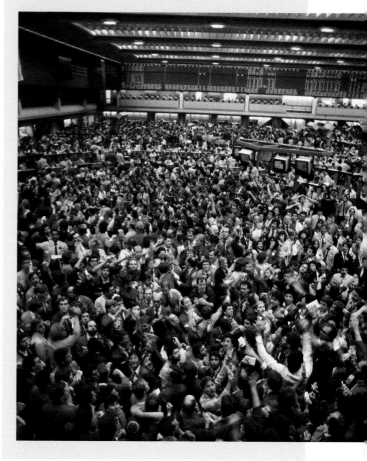

who had recently separated or divorced from their spouses. Taking periodic blood samples, they found that certain immune functions of these women were "significantly poorer," even after a year, than were the immune functions of well-matched women in the same community who were still married. And among those married women, researchers found that those who felt they had a good marriage had stronger immune responses.

FALLING DOWN ON THE JOB

So if your marriage is teetering, your immune system could be tottering. You might well ask whether all those millions of immune cells don't have something better to do than worry about marital harmony and discord.

Well, yes, they do. Researchers have found that the immune system seems to respond to all kinds of stresses and strains that are the human lot. Like unemployment.

One Swedish study followed the lives of a number of unemployed women and found that their bank accounts were not the only thing that plummeted. Their immune systems, compared to their employed counterparts', also took a nosedive. After nine months of unemployment, the women's lymphocytes, immune cells responsible for protecting the body from viral attack, still showed depressed functioning.

Nor have the Glasers at Ohio State University confined their research to marital strife. In another study, they looked at the immune systems of family members caring for people with Alzheimer's disease. They found that the chronic stress has an impact on the immune system.

Caregivers had "significantly lower percentages" of total T-lymphocytes and helper T-lymphocytes in their blood than did their peers. Again, these immune cells play an important role in preventing infection and disease.

THE DISTRESS OF STRESS

The daily stresses of professional life have also come under scrutiny.

Researchers at the University of Toronto investigated the role of acute and chronic stress in the lives of accountants. They gave the accountants tests to measure their "psychological distress, personality, behavioral style and coping strategies." They also looked at a number of immune functions in their blood.

Accountants, not surprisingly, proved to be more stressed at income tax time. Researchers concluded that data from the study "suggest that chronic occupational stress may increase susceptibility to disease."

Even something as mundane as taking an exam can show up in the immune system. A study at Ohio State University drew two blood samples from 75 first-year medical students. One sample was taken a month before their final examination and the second on the first day of the finals. Natural killer cell activity in the students declined "significantly" on the day of the exam.

In the same study, students who showed high stress in their lives or who reported being lonely also had slower natural killer cells than did their peers.

What's going on here? What does it all mean?

LIFE ISN'T A TEST TUBE

"The clinical applications right now are probably not that much different than before we understood some of these underlying neuroimmunological mechanisms," says Dr. Sobel. "We still say to people, 'It's probably a good idea to maintain a positive attitude. It's probably a good idea to relax and manage stress a little bit better so it's less taxing on you.'

"What recent research has done is to add weight to why people should follow certain practices—whether it's relaxing more, managing stress, laughing more or being more involved with other people. One additional reason people can give themselves now is, 'It bolsters my immune system.'"

Some researchers are concerned that in the enthusiasm to find new mental treatments for physical disease, science may be getting pushed aside.

"In terms of our current knowledge, we're more

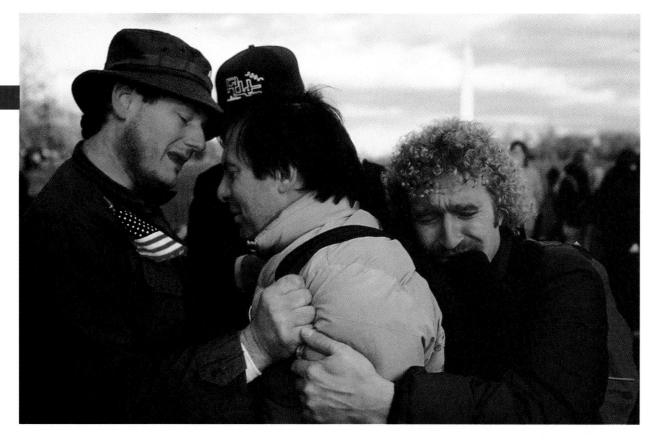

at the fact-gathering stages than at the explanatory stage. I would say we're approaching square two maybe, but we haven't really left square one," says Robert Ader, Ph.D., director of the Division of Behavioral and Psychosocial Medicine at the University of Rochester.

Dr. Ader, a pioneer in the field, is the man who coined the term *psychoneuroimmunology.* Although he urges caution, his own work in conditioning the immune systems of experimental animals is causing a good deal of excitement. If animals can learn to alter their immune response, the implication is that people can, too.

Someday this may happen, Dr. Ader agrees, but the science has to happen before the clinical applications can follow.

"Psychological functioning *can* have an influence on the development, susceptibility and progression of a disease," he says. "Disease is an extremely complicated process that involves the entire organism. There *is* no separation of mind and body.

"Miraculous cures, spontaneous remission—those are real phenomena that are buried under the rug because we have no mechanistic explanation for them in a mechanistic society. That does not make

Veterans who gather at the Vietnam Veterans Memorial in Washington, D.C., express grief that in some cases has festered for years. Apparently, the agony of grief penetrates all the way to the cellular level. Researchers have found that grief and certain other negative emotions suppress some functions of the immune system.

the phenomena any less real, but they are very difficult to study."

The potential role of psychoneuroimmunologic interactions in the spontaneous remission of cancer, for example, may take a while to figure out. But while scientists haven't yet put miracles into test tubes to study, real doctors in real hospitals aren't waiting. They are already trying out all kinds of methods to tap into the mind's healing potential.

Techniques like relaxation training, self-hypnosis, imagery, visualization and meditation are showing up in hospital settings and doctors' offices. Even laughter is now official. Some hospitals are providing patients with "laughmobiles"—carts full of humorous books, cassette tapes, cartoons and toys. Medical schools are looking into adding humor to the curriculum. Nurses are polishing up on jokes.

STRESS-FIGHTING TECHNIQUES

You don't have to visit a doctor's office to encourage your mind to boost your immunity. Stress-fighting techniques like self-hypnosis, progressive relaxation and imagery can all be done at home. And if you *are* under a doctor's care, you can work on your attitude at the same time you follow whatever medical advice he or she may give you. (Just don't be surprised if you get a prescription for laughter along with your pills.)

Here are a number of stress-fighting techniques recommended by experts in the field.

Relaxation. Select a relaxation technique that works for you—some form of meditation, even just sitting with your eyes closed and listening to music— and use it every day.

Exercise. Exercise increases your level of endorphins, the brain's morphinelike substances that create euphoria. With regular exercise you'll feel less tense and more positive.

Cognitive restructuring. A fancy term that simply means being aware of your own inner dialogue and fixing it when necessary. The idea is to watch for negative self-put-downs ("Oh, you dummy, why are you so stupid?") and to talk to yourself nicely instead.

Cutting back on caffeine. Coffee, tea, colas— any beverages that contain caffeine—can add to your stress levels if you overindulge. Try herb teas instead.

Self-awareness. Learn to recognize the physical signs of stress in yourself—clenched jaw, tight neck and shoulder muscles, rapid heartbeat, churning stomach—and pause to take a few deep breaths when you feel stress coming on.

Crying. Go ahead if you feel like crying. Let the tears flow. Experts say that crying discharges tension, provides an emotional release and even helps restore chemical balance to the body.

Sleeping. Getting enough sleep helps your immune system deal with stress.

Love. Love yourself and cultivate your friendships and family relationships. Experts say that learning to express your feelings is vital for your health.

Counseling. If you find yourself unable to cope with stressful situations in your life, seek professional counseling to defuse the stress before it does its damage.

Imagery. On the other hand, you might want to color yourself well. Dust the cobwebs off those mental pictures of perfect health and breathe new life into them.

Many doctors and researchers maintain that what you picture in your mind can have either a detrimental or a healing impact on the body, depending upon whether what you see is negative or positive. At some cancer treatment centers, patients are even taught to visualize their immune cells routing out the cancer and defeating it. Although such treatment is still highly controversial, there have been reports of spectacular successes.

And, if stress, tension and the traumas of daily living do indeed have a debilitating effect on the immune system, you should be interested in any tool that helps you cope. Mental imagery is such a tool.

"It certainly can be used in the reduction of fear and worry, by mentally rehearsing what might happen in a given situation. The nervous system does not distinguish between a real event and what's imagined. If you imagine Thanksgiving dinner vividly enough, you're going to salivate," says Neil Fiore, Ph.D., psychologist and author of *The Road Back to Health.*

Most people already know how to do mental imagery. The problem is that they do "negative rehearsals" of bad things that might happen in their lives, says Dr. Fiore. That's what you are doing when you worry—running negative images through your mind.

Dr. Fiore recommends seizing control of your already highly evolved capacity to make mental images and using it for your health. Try running positive images through your mind. Instead of stressing yourself out, you'll be doing your body a favor.

If positive images elude you, try visualizing to music. Researchers at Southern Methodist University in Dallas, Texas, have found that music seems to enhance the effects of mental imagery. Music thera-

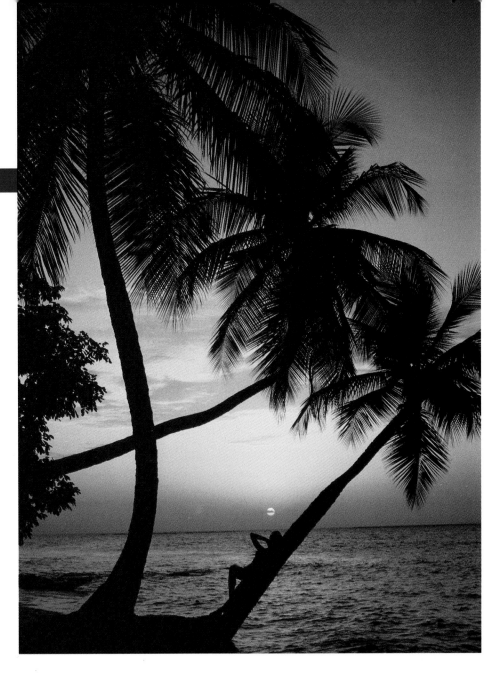

Just can't manage a two-week getaway this year? Your immune system may need it more than you do, but don't panic. Some immune system functions are so responsive to R&R that apparently even a 5-minute mental vacation can yield benefits. Some researchers recommend combining deep relaxation with an inner visualization of your favorite vacation place. Five minutes "at the beach" and your disease-fighting cells should be back in the swim.

pist Mark Rider, working with psychologist Jeanne Achterberg, Ph.D., taught people to form mental images of specific cells in their immune systems increasing in number. The exercises were done while listening to specially composed "entrainment" music. The specific immune cells visualized were indeed the only ones to increase significantly.

A pleasant way to experience positive mental imagery is to select a relaxing place, such as a mountain scene, and visit it in your mind. Do it while listening to music that soothes you, says Rider.

"Music has most of its effects on human beings through imagery. Music conjures up pictures and emotions," he says. "The music should be nonvocal and without a strong beat."

Progressive relaxation. Still tense? Stressed out?

Slip into something comfortable—a frame of mind that will relax and benefit your body.

A good way to start working on either an imagery exercise or something as involved as self-hypnosis is with tailor-made relaxation techniques. And something like progressive relaxation is good for you all by itself.

In fact, some clinicians make very little distinction between progressive relaxation and self-hypnosis. William Coe, Ph.D., president of the Psychological Hypnosis Division of the American Psychological Association, says he uses the terms interchangeably, depending upon whether a client is afraid of the idea of hypnosis or attracted to it.

Here is the progressive relaxation technique that Dr. Coe has shared with numerous clients.

Sit back. Take a couple of nice deep breaths. Close your eyes and let your body get very heavy. Now focus all your attention on your left foot. Imagine the muscles going loose. Feel the individual toes and imagine the muscles relaxing.

Now focus on your left calf and do the same thing. Feel it relaxing. Move up your left leg, then the right, then the left arm and the right arm. Finally concentrate on the trunk, the neck and the head. The whole process takes about 20 minutes, and by the end of that time your body should be completely relaxed.

"It's easier to start with just your foot than it is to try to relax your whole body. But with practice, you can relax the whole body in about a minute," says Dr. Coe.

Another progressive relaxation technique calls for tensing each body part before relaxing it. This gives you practice in sensing the difference between tension and relaxation.

For most people, progressive relaxation takes practice. You can't try it just once and dismiss it, because the relaxation gets deeper and the benefits greater the more you practice.

"It's like saying, 'I want to play the piano.' If I say 'Well, here, play the piano. Punch those keys,' people aren't going to be able to make music at first. People look at relaxation as something they can just *get*. But it's more like learning to read or write. It's a skill, and as you practice you get better and better at it," says Dr. Coe.

Relaxation skills can be an important part of any type of healing. "You relax the mind and body so there's less stress and more energy for healing. In any healing, relaxation makes more energy available to the inner wisdom of the body," says Dr. Fiore.

By "inner wisdom," he means the body's innate ability to heal itself, "the body's tendency to always go toward health and healing."

Self-hypnosis. Self-hypnosis is another tool for healing. It is one more servant that you can call on when you're working on your positive attitude and coping with life's daily stresses.

Dr. Fiore, who is president of the Northern California Society of Clinical Hypnosis, makes a clear-cut distinction between relaxation and self-hypnosis.

"The main difference is that hypnosis is for a purpose or a goal," he says. "It's more directed. With meditation and relaxation, on the other hand, I'm just emptying my mind. I'm letting go.

"Self-hypnosis is an altered state of consciousness, just like meditation, praying or any one of a number of altered states of consciousness. The difference is that hypnosis (ironically enough), given the popular definition of it, is consciously controlled for a specific goal or purpose." In self-hypnosis, the one doing the conscious controlling is you.

Deep relaxation is a prerequisite for self-hypnosis. Once you reach the relaxed state, you make suggestions to yourself either in the form of images or statements. When you are relaxed and feel safe, the body and mind are open and will accept the pictures and words that you give it.

"Hypnosis has been used for pain control, bladder control, dilation of the blood vessels to warm the extremities and constriction of the blood vessels to stop bleeding. It's really a tool for communicating with your body in a language that it understands," says Dr. Fiore.

"Hypnosis is used in burn centers for pain control. It's often used in surgery so people need less anesthesia or even none at all. It's often used in childbirth. It's an extremely powerful tool. Given the world we live in, it's remarkable to me that people can function without some form of hypnosis, relaxation or imagery every day."

If you're interested in learning the powerful techniques of self-hypnosis, a good way to start is by practicing progressive relaxation or some form of meditation. "I've found that people who have done transcendental meditation or *any* kind of meditation are very good at using self-hypnosis. They already know what it feels like to get into that state of mind, and they can access it very readily," says Dr. Fiore.

He also recommends yogic breathing or deep-

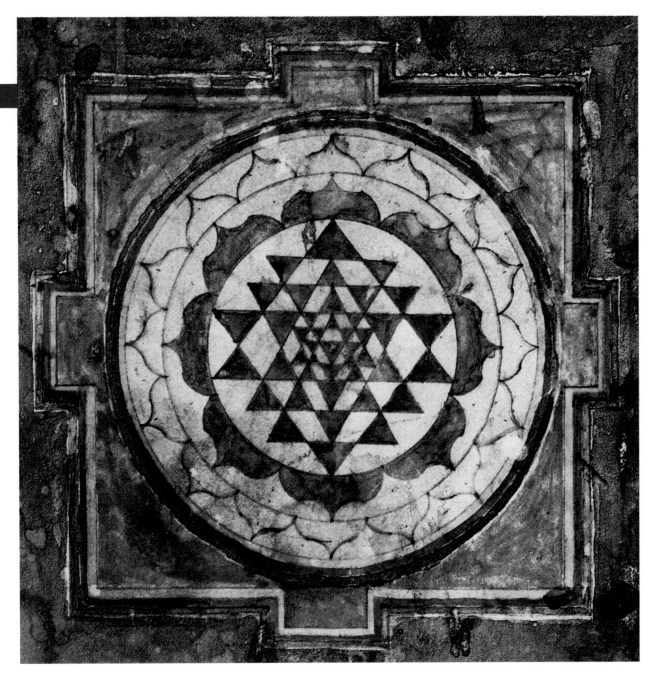

breathing exercises. Slow the breath down to 12 breaths a minute, holding each breath for a moment before exhaling slowly and completely. Even a minute of practice helps the body relax.

If the techniques of progressive relaxation, imagery or self-hypnosis elude you but you still feel that you might benefit from them, seek the help of a professional.

You might ask your personal physician or your local medical society to recommend someone who can train you to relieve stress.

Relaxation and meditation techniques to help the immune system are nothing new. The *sri yantra*—an ancient Hindu symbol of creation—is used by yogis as a visual focus for many different types of meditation, among them one that supposedly helps the body resist disease. Such meditations are thousands of years old, according to Pandit Ramjami Tigunait, Ph.D., a member of the faculty of the Himalayan Institute of Yoga in Honesdale, Pennsylvania. You shouldn't expect instant results, however. Proper use of the *sri yantra* involves many years of instruction and study, says Dr. Tigunait.

NUTRITION AND IMMUNITY

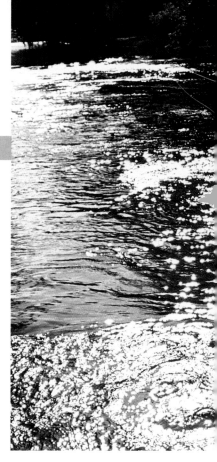

Imagine you're the mess hall sergeant in charge of feeding a fighting army. What do you put on the menu? Coffee and a Danish for breakfast? Low-cal diet shakes for lunch? Chips and soda for dinner? Of course not. A steady diet like that and the troops would soon be drained of the energy they need to square off against the enemy at the front line.

Well, you *are* in charge of nourishing an army—the legions of lymphocytes and other white blood cells that engage in daily hand-to-hand combat with body-invading bacteria, viruses, tumor cells, toxins and other enemies. And scientists are discovering that what you put on your plate could mean the difference between helping your body win the war on infection and losing out to colds, flu or maybe even more serious diseases like cancer.

"Our ability to fight an infection depends on how well our immune system functions," says Brian Morgan, Ph.D., assistant professor of human nutrition at Columbia University College of Physicians and Surgeons. "Any nutritional deficiencies can seriously impair the various components of the body's immune system."

Notice that Dr. Morgan is talking about nutritional *deficiencies*—severe shortages of essential nutrients. For example, studies show that malnourished children who subsist on meager bowls of rice have depleted immune defenses. Their thymus glands (the "command headquarters" where infection-fighting cells are made) shrink and they have fewer antibodies (the custom-made molecules that latch onto enemy invaders).

But Dr. Morgan isn't only talking about famine victims. "We're discovering," he explains, "that the 'undernourished'—those who lack one or more nutrients, such as dieters, fast-food fans, older folks—may also have impaired immune systems."

Neglect to eat your vegetables and other vitamin A-rich foods, for example, and you may be more susceptible to a bout with an infection in your respi-

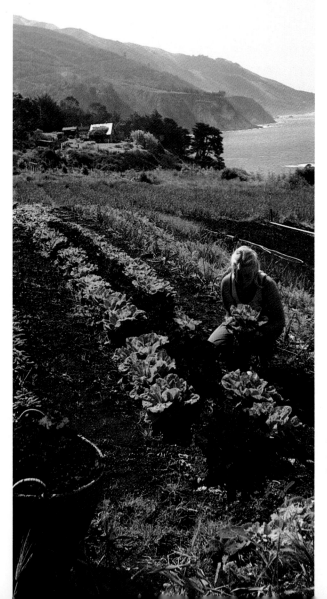

Freshly picked leafy greens make dazzling salads and play an impressive role in fortifying the immune system. They're bursting with vitamins A and C and minerals, nutrients that help your body manufacture protective white blood cells.

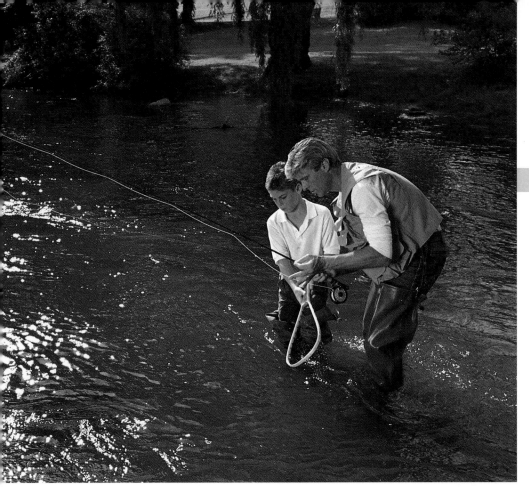

It's never too early to start instilling good eating habits for lifelong health. A diet rich in fresh fish, for example, boosts the immune system and can provide an important hedge against infections.

ratory tract or other mucus-lined area. Studies indicate that vitamin A helps the epithelial cells secrete mucus, which in turn helps defend against microorganisms.

Or leave out vitamin B-rich foods like bread and cereals, and your body may not muster foot

Make it a point to stop regularly at your local produce stand. Feasting on a variety of fruits and vegetables could be one of the best ways to protect yourself from illness.

soldiers—T-lymphocyte cells—to effectively fight that flu bug going around.

Pass up the citrus fruits (an important source of vitamin C) and you may have less effective macrophage cells to patrol your bloodstream and engulf tumor cells.

Even too little seafood (rich in zinc) may mean less of the thymic hormone that dispatches the "Green Berets"—the natural killer cells that finish off virulent viruses.

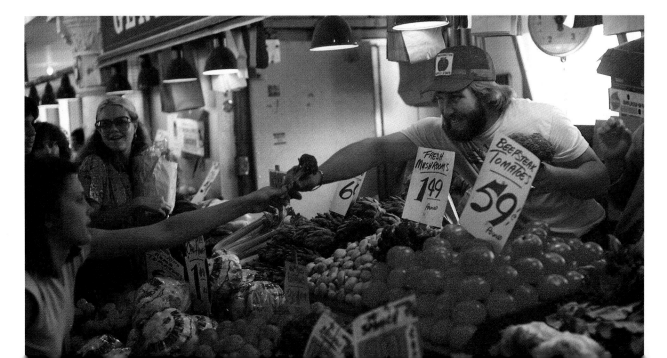

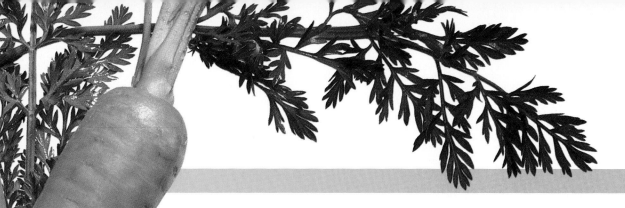

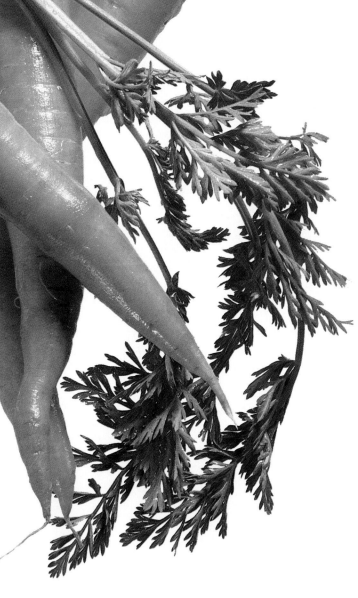

So how do you plan your menu to keep the immune army in infection-fighting shape? "Think balance," says Dr. Morgan. "Choose foods low in fat, high in fiber and full of vitamins and minerals."

Here's a final important fact before we introduce you to the individual nutrients. In the "mess hall line," the immune troops get fed *after* the brain, nervous system and other key body components. So make every meal count.

VITAMIN A

How many times have you done this? You're out to dinner and when your entrée arrives, you flick off the parsley sprigs, shove those jagged carrot slices to the side—and would as soon eat the Romaine lettuce as the plate. Or, at the wine and cheese party, you're so busy sampling the vino that you completely forget about the cheese.

If that's your routine, think about changing it. These foods have more important work to do than just dress up a party tray or the chef's special. They all supply vitamin A, which helps fortify your body's first line of defense—the top layers of your skin.

Vitamin A maintains the integrity of your skin so that microorganisms can't penetrate. But if you pass up those vitamin A-rich foods too many times, your skin can become dry and full of cracks—tiny portals for infections.

A second way that vitamin A keeps invaders at arm's length is by promoting the rapid turnover of the epithelial cells lining the mouth, lungs, bladder, stomach, intestines, cervix and even the retina of the eyes. An important function of some epithelial cells is to secrete protective mucus.

"A vitamin A deficiency may slow epithelial cell production and dry up the mucous membranes," says Susan Smith, Ph.D., research fellow in the Department of Physiology and Biophysics, Harvard Medical School. That may be why people who have cancer of the mouth, throat or lung have been shown to also have low levels of vitamin A in their blood.

But this knowledge about vitamin A is more than

Here's a new twist to an old idea: "A carrot a day keeps disease away." Studies have shown that people who eat carrots (or other yellow-orange foods) have less cancer.

a warning against deficiency. Scientists have found that adding even a small amount of extra vitamin A to the diet could help fortify the mucosal defense mechanism in areas like the respiratory tract.

Australian researchers at the University of Adelaide studied 147 preschool children who were prone to respiratory infections like bronchitis. They gave one group 450 international units of supplemental vitamin A. (That's the equivalent of half a carrot or a small piece of cheese). The other group was given a fake supplement (placebo). After 11 months, the children who took the supplements had experienced 19 percent fewer episodes of respiratory distress than their counterparts not receiving extra vitamin A.

These preliminary results may be heartening to parents who know too well that respiratory infections often circulate among kids at a day care center or school faster than a new toy. Perhaps, suggest the researchers, getting the children to eat more cheese could limit the contagion.

Asleep at the Switch

Infections are persistent. If there's a chance to get past your skin's surface, they will. What happens

A parsley sprig isn't just a good-looking garnish; it could be a real heavyweight in defending your body against infections because it's a rich source of vitamin A.

then? Your T-lymphocyte cells—the cells produced by the thymus gland—multiply their ranks. Then you notice redness and swelling, indicating that your immune system has gone into battle.

But without vitamin A, there may be no redness, no swelling, no T-cell victory over the enemy invaders. Recently, Dr. Smith and her colleagues looked at what happened when the offspring of rats who were fed a balanced diet except for an absence of vitamin A were injected with a foreign protein just under their skin. The rats showed only a fourth of the normal swelling.

It appears, says Dr. Smith, that "vitamin A acts as a switch." It turns on the T-cells, which in turn summon the backup defense of antibodies, the specialized lobsterlike molecules that grab onto certain invaders and deactivate them. "With a vitamin A deficiency, this switch doesn't get thrown."

In lab animals, at least, the T-cell activity may be restored with high doses of vitamin A. But in humans, notes Dr. Smith, high doses of retinol, the kind of vitamin A found in supplements as well as in liver

The sweet, odd-shaped papaya may be a boon to your immune system. Its sunshine yellow color comes from beta-carotene, a nutrient that scientists have found stimulates infection-fighting macrophages.

and cheese, can be toxic and may even backfire in the immune system.

Why Beta May Be Best

But there's another kind of vitamin A—beta-carotene. It's found in carrots and other yellow-orange foods and some leafy green ones, too. It may be safer—and a superior immune booster.

Retinol can be risky because it's stored in the liver, where a buildup can become toxic. But beta-carotene is stored in the skin, and the worst symptom of excess seems to be a yellow-orange color.

But the best thing about beta-carotene is that it appears to play a positive role against some types of cancer.

Studies from scientists around the world show that those who eat more foods rich in beta-carotene seem to have less cancer. Italian researchers, for example, compared the diets of 191 women with cervical cancer to the same number of healthy women. They discovered that those who got more vitamin A from foods high in beta-carotene had a reduced risk of cancer. They found no such benefit among those who merely consumed retinol-rich foods like milk, meat and cheese.

How might beta-carotene offer protection from tumors? First, it guards cell membranes against corrosive oxidation damage, which occurs when your body metabolizes fat or is exposed to environmental toxins.

But should tumor cells actually arise, beta-carotene may be able to stop them. "Lab studies show that this nutrient stimulates the macrophages,"

says Ronald Ross Watson, Ph.D., of the University of Arizona School of Medicine. These are the large cells that search out tumors, engulf them and zap them with a lethal chemical.

Could eating cantaloupe stave off other problems? "At this point," Dr. Watson says, "we believe that beta-carotene may very well decrease the risk of certain diseases."

In one report, researchers at the Albert Einstein College of Medicine added beta-carotene to human cells in test tubes. They found an increase in immune activity against *Candida albicans*, a bacterial yeast infection.

Currently, there's no Recommended Dietary Allowance (RDA) set for beta-carotene. (For adult males, the RDA for all forms of vitamin A combined is 5,000 international units daily; for women, it's 4,000 international units.) But it's a good idea to eat a variety of vitamin A foods anyway, says Dr. Watson, to get the maximum immune benefits. So, drink your milk for retinol, eat your broccoli for beta-carotene and remember those garnishes aren't just good-looking—they're good for you, too.

FOLATE

If you're not a fan of salads, you could be missing out on something special. Leafy greens contain folate, a B vitamin that has been shown to be a powerful infection fighter.

Even if you do eat some greens now and then, though, your body still might be deficient in folate. Taking oral contraceptives or drinking alcohol could mean less folate in your system. Even growing older can interfere. That may be one reason why the elderly are more prone to infectious diseases, especially pneumonia.

Folate is needed to make special white blood cells such as the macrophages, the large lymphocytes that surround and eat infectious organisms. When folate is lacking, studies have found, these defenders may decrease in number or effectiveness.

"When one realizes that up to one-third of all

premenopausal women in America have less than optimal intakes of folate, these effects could actually be widespread," says Dr. Morgan.

The flip side of these studies is more encouraging. When people with lowered immune responses were given additional folate, their cells were able to kill off bacteria.

Folate may also help strengthen cell membranes and guard them against mutation. When women with Pap smears revealing abnormal cervical cells were given high doses of folate, the abnormalities disappeared.

VITAMIN B₆

"One look into the shopping carts of older folks and you can often tell what shape their immune systems might be in," says Lorraine Miller, Ph.D., professor of food and nutrition at Oregon State University. "They usually aren't buying soda and chips, but they may be loading up on white bread and cottage cheese."

What's so wrong with that? Just that they may be passing up whole grain breads, red meat and good sources of vitamin B₆. And that, she says, is no way to feed your immune system. White blood cells need B₆ to produce antibodies, and the thymus gland requires it to produce lymphocytes.

A study by Dr. Miller demonstrates just how important this vitamin is for older people. She and her colleagues looked at 15 persons aged 6 to 81 who were eating their normal diets. They gave one group 50 milligrams per day of supplemental pyridoxine (another name for B₆) while the other group got a look-alike pill. After two months, the B₆ group showed increased lymphocyte proliferation.

Other studies underscore B₆'s role as an infection fighter. When researchers at Loma Linda University in California fed mice very high doses of B₆, the animals showed higher immune responses and slower tumor growth. But there was one more intriguing finding, notes Daila Gridley, Ph.D., assistant professor of microbiology and immunology.

Hors d'oeuvres anyone? That paté on the party tray is rich in B vitamins that can increase lymphocyte cell activity.

"B₆ appeared to enhance the T-helper cells," Dr. Gridley explains. T-helper cells are the lymphocytes that help trigger other immune responses and the cells that are often destroyed by the human immune virus (HIV) in AIDS patients.

That's not to suggest that B₆ in high doses is the answer to AIDS—or any other disease. "Doses over 50 milligrams could damage the nervous system," warns Dr. Gridley.

Still, most of us barely get a third of the RDA, says Terry D. Shultz, Ph.D., assistant professor of biochemistry at Loma Linda University. (The RDA is 2 milligrams.) His advice? Avoid foods made from refined grains (which lose their B₆ in the milling process) and fill your shopping cart with meats, kidney beans, black-eyed peas, bananas, whole grain breads and other B₆-rich foods.

PANTOTHENATE

Although it's a B vitamin, it doesn't have an RDA. Yet pantothenate, or pantothenic acid, is added to many vitamin supplements, and even cereals are fortified with it.

Until recently, though, there has been very little evidence to demonstrate the importance of pantothenate in the body. Won O. Song, Ph.D., assistant professor of human nutrition at Michigan State University hopes her studies will highlight this nutrient's special role in the immune system.

In experiments with rats, Dr. Song found that a deficiency of pantothenate causes a decrease in antibodies, the Y-shaped infection fighters that grab onto specific antigens with lobsterlike claws. Dr. Song's next step is to test the hypothesis that a pantothenate deficiency can increase gastrointestinal infections. "We'll be measuring the antibody responses at the gut level in both humans and animals," Dr. Song says.

If the connection tests out, an RDA may finally be established for pantothenate. In the meantime, you can hedge your bets by including whole wheat bread, wheat germ, liver and other good sources of this nutrient in your diet regularly.

VITAMIN B$_{12}$

This vitamin may also play a part in keeping the immune system vital. Researchers have observed that in patients with pernicious anemia, a disease caused by a lack of B$_{12}$, the bacteria-eating phagocytes are less active.

B$_{12}$ may also help keep tumors from destroying cells. One researcher took vitamin B$_{12}$, mixed it with vitamin C and fed this cocktail to tumor cells. The membranes of the malignant cells were altered so that special tumor-killing cells could more easily recognize them and complete their mission.

You can get B$_{12}$ from foods like meat, eggs and cheese.

VITAMIN C

While it may not be as comforting as a steamy bowl of chicken soup, many people think that taking lots of this nutrient can help fight sneezes, coughs and other ravages of winter.

The fact is, scientists have been unsuccessful at proving that vitamin C can prevent, or cure, the common cold. But some studies do point to a reduction of severe cold symptoms in those taking extra vitamin C.

And the latest research is definitely onto something very important regarding vitamin C's role in

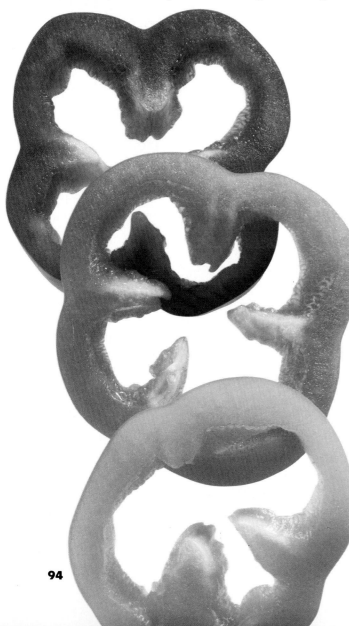

Bell peppers are loaded with vitamin C, which may help keep you infection-free.

the immune system. Benjamin Siegel, Ph.D., professor of pathology at the Oregon Health Sciences University in Portland, found that vitamin C stimulates the production of interferon, a chemical so named because it "interferes" with the reproduction of viruses.

It works like this. When a virus invades, cells secrete interferon, which acts as a kind of biochemical Paul Revere, warning neighboring cells about the viral invasion. These cells then take up arms and keep the virus from spreading.

Interferon has another mission, too. It triggers tumor destruction. When Dr. Siegel put 250 milligrams of vitamin C daily in the drinking water of mice, he found that the level of interferon in their blood increased and that their susceptibility to leukemia, a kind of blood cancer, was reduced. In this case, Dr. Siegel explains, interferon triggered the production of natural killer cells, which target and destroy tumors.

It may turn out that vitamin C could even play a role against one of the deadliest diseases—AIDS. Vitamin C activates interleukin-1, the messenger hormone that stimulates a type of lymphocyte called the T-helper cell. These helpers in turn send signals to antibodies, which then spring into action against tumors. "In AIDS patients, the T-helper cell is destroyed by the human immune virus," Dr. Siegel says. "Possibly, vitamin C may help enhance immunocompetence in people."

At this point, there are no human studies that clearly demonstrate that vitamin C can prevent anything as serious as AIDS or as minor as the common cold. Still, test-tube findings like the one at the University of Florida are encouraging. There, elderly volunteers were given 2 grams (2,000 milligrams) of vitamin C daily for three weeks. When their cells were analyzed, they showed enhanced lymphocyte proliferation. (Never take more than the RDA of vitamin C or any other nutrient without the approval and supervision of your doctor.)

You don't have to wait for the final word—or

Van Gogh appreciated the sunflower for its striking beauty. Now scientists are learning that the vitamin E in this stately plant's seeds may help keep infection-fighting T-cell production switched on.

wintertime—to boost your intake of vitamin C-rich foods. Citrus fruit and juices are excellent sources. Or try more exotic fruits like papaya or kiwi. Top your burger with green peppers. And order a baked potato the next time you visit the drive-up window.

VITAMIN E

When researcher Jeffrey Blumberg, Ph.D., assistant director of the USDA/Tufts Nutrition Center, gave aged mice very high doses of vitamin E supplements, he discovered that it enhanced immune responses.

Vitamin E appears to work like this, explains

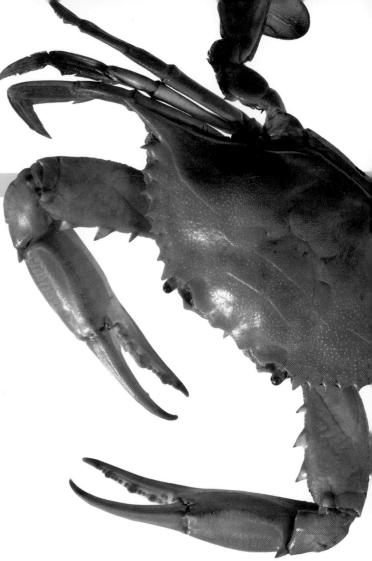

Dr. Blumberg. "Your immune system requires a prostaglandin hormone, called E_2, in order to work correctly. E_2 acts as a kind of negative regulator—it turns off the production of T-lymphocytes.

"When we age, though, E_2 appears to increase, further suppressing the immune response. That's where vitamin E comes in—it retards E_2 production. In other words, it turns the off switch back on."

Dr. Blumberg hopes to soon release the results of another study involving the immune responses of human volunteers who were supplemented with vitamin E.

Meanwhile, other studies have looked at vitamin E's ability to protect cells. One experiment showed that rats given high doses of vitamin E before exposure to air pollutants suffered much less cell damage in their lungs. And in a British study, women with the lowest levels of vitamin E were found to have a risk of breast cancer five times higher than that of women with the highest levels.

Both breast cancer and damage from air pollution may be caused by free radicals, molecules that destroy cell membranes by oxidizing them—a kind of vicious internal rust.

"Mother Nature recognized that free radical damage could cut cells in their prime, so she gave us natural antioxidants like vitamin E that quench free radicals," says Dr. Blumberg. "They soak up the oxidizing products so they cannot harm your cells."

More studies are needed to uncover all the ways vitamin E may prevent the age-regulated decline in our immune systems. But outstanding food sources of vitamin E are available right now. Try adding some wheat germ to your baked goods. One tablespoon provides 37 international units of vitamin E—7 units over the RDA. You can also toss sunflower seeds in your salads, and drizzle on some safflower oil for even more vitamin E.

IRON

Iron is more than just a builder of healthy blood. White blood cells—the backbone of the immune system—need this mineral just as much as the energy-pumping red blood cells. Why? Because iron makes hemoglobin, the protein that carries oxygen to *all* cells.

A healthy supply of oxygen, for example, enables the phagocyte immune cells to engulf an invading bacterium and kill it with a deadly chemical. "If you don't have enough iron, you could fall prey to a

Savory steamed crab is a good source of iron, a mineral that may protect you against viruses and other infectious organisms.

host of garden-variety bacterial infections, especially those in the gastrointestinal tract," explains Adria Rothman Sherman, Ph.D., chairperson of the Department of Home Economics at Rutgers University.

Low iron levels may also mean a weak defense against viruses.

Dr. Sherman compared iron-deficient rat pups with pups fed normal diets, and then injected them both with a virus. The iron-deficient rats had less natural killer activity against the virus. These killer cells are the immune system's special tactical unit; they hunt down tumor cells and shoot them with a disintegrating chemical.

If your body is low in iron, Dr. Sherman found, you may also have less of the messenger hormone called interleukin-1. It's interleukin's job to signal the T-cells, which in turn dispatch the natural killer cells to destroy the enemy.

"All this becomes quite significant when you consider that 20 percent of adult women in the United States are not getting enough iron," notes Dr. Sherman. "Women should try to get the RDA of 18 milligrams daily." But don't overdo it on iron, especially if you already have a bacterial infection. It seems that bacteria thrive on iron overload.

Your best bet is to eat iron-rich foods. Add turkey dark meat to your salad or include some navy beans in that casserole you're baking. You can further enhance your iron absorption by serving vitamin C-rich foods with your meals. And use iron cookware when you can; studies show a minimal amount of the mineral actually migrates to the food.

ZINC

Next birthday, forget the cake; ask for oysters. These odd-shaped mollusks are exceptionally rich sources of zinc. And that mineral, say experts, may help your immune system provide you with many birthdays to come.

How did scientists come to that discovery? For openers, they observed that older people often have a shrunken thymus gland. (That's the organ where

Pearls are beautiful, but the real gem inside these tasty oysters is zinc. This mineral helps keep the thymus gland producing T-cells.

infection-fighting T-cells are produced.) The few T-cells that do get made are often too weak to rally against infections.

Then lab experiments like the one at the Veterans Administration Medical Center in Los Angeles began to reveal something very interesting. When rats were fed zinc-deprived diets, their immune systems started to resemble the withered systems found in humans.

Further experiments showed that a lack of zinc prevented a thymic hormone from kicking in. And with only a trickle of the hormone, the T-cells can't multiply or summon the aid of the natural killer cells.

"We're learning that zinc is crucial to so many parts of the immune system and that a lack of it becomes critical," says Susanna Cunningham-Rundles, Ph.D., associate professor of immunology at New York Hospital/Cornell Medical Center.

Yet a lack of zinc is commonplace among the elderly. Could adding zinc put new life into a sagging immune system? Researchers at the University of Florida studied more than 200 people aged 60 and over, 22 of whom had low-functioning immune systems. When a small group of them were given zinc supplements for four weeks, their resistance to antigens increased. And at the University of California in San Diego, 17 people aged 66 to 85 were given zinc supplements. After three months, they had

Next time you're yearning for a chewy treat, try a handful of dried apricots. They contain copper, which may help boost the infection-fighting white blood cells. Or, try snacking on selenium-rich mushrooms.

increased lymphocytes and antibodies.

Interestingly, other studies show that zinc given in doses many times the RDA of 15 milligrams *depresses* the immune system.

You can't go wrong, though, getting your supply of zinc from seafood, beef, pumpkin seeds and other food sources. And don't wait until your next birthday. Zinc isn't stored in the body, so it must be replenished daily.

SELENIUM

Forget pesticides. In parts of China the farmers spray *selenium* on their crops.

It's part of a public health program, because the Chinese know that if the soil is selenium-deficient, people have higher rates of cancer, especially liver cancer. And where selenium soil levels are high, people have lower rates of some cancers, including stomach and esophageal cancer.

Selenium may protect against cancer because it's found in an enzyme called glutathione peroxide (GSH-Px). GSH-Px helps stop the formation of free radicals, chemicals that can speed tumor formation. Researchers at the Univesity of Miami School of Medicine found that cancer patients in selenium-poor regions had low levels of GSH-Px in their blood.

Even if tumors do form, there's some evidence that selenium may help them disappear. Studies

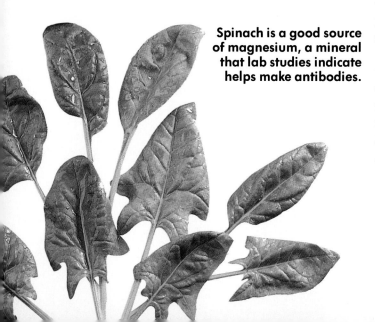

Spinach is a good source of magnesium, a mineral that lab studies indicate helps make antibodies.

have shown a regression of tumors in lab animals fed selenium. "What appears to be happening is that selenium accelerates the killing activity of phagocytes," says Lidia Kiremidjian-Schumacher, Ph.D., professor of oral medicine and pathology at New York University College of Dentistry. These immune cells devour tumor cells.

Phagocytes also fight other foreign invaders such as viruses and bacteria. That's why cows supplemented with selenium were able to fight off bacterial disease. And selenium-rich diets helped mice resist pneumonia.

Dr. Kiremidjian-Schumacher says that adequate body levels of selenium may prevent tumors and other diseases. That's not to suggest you should pump up your immune system by loading up on selenium supplements, however. Low doses of selenium supplements appear to stimulate the immune system, but high doses may actually suppress it.

But you should make sure your diet is normal. "It's up to each of us to make sure we get enough selenium in our own diets," says Dr. Kiremidjian-Schumacher. The best way to do that is to choose selenium-rich foods like fresh meats and seafood, especially shellfish. Mushrooms, radishes, carrots and cabbage are also good sources of selenium. The selenium content of most other fruits and vegetables is much lower and more likely to depend upon where they are grown.

MAGNESIUM

Magnesium is an essential mineral that, in animals at least, clearly plays an important role in making infection-fighting white blood cells. When mice drank water with low magnesium levels, they were shown to have suppressed levels of antibodies.

It's premature to say just what happens to the

human immune system when magnesium deficiency occurs, cautions Carl Keen, Ph.D., associate professor of nutrition and internal medicine at the University of California at Davis.

Still, for this and other reasons (like heart health), it's a good idea to make sure you get enough magnesium. You may not know how much is in your water. (Hard water usually has more than soft water.) But you can make sure you get it in your diet if you include foods like nuts, soybeans and whole grain bread.

COPPER

One indication that copper may be related to immunity is that people who have Menkes syndrome—a hereditary disease characterized by kinky hair and low blood levels of copper—often die of pneumonia or other infections.

Another clue: Where forage crops are low in copper, cattle and sheep have decreased protection against viral and bacterial diseases.

Research with lab animals is providing more

Red cabbage contains selenium, a mineral that's been shown to accelerate the germ-killing activity of phagocytes.

insights into copper's role. Scientists at Oregon State University looked at rats who were marginally deficient in copper. They found that they had smaller thymus glands as well as fewer T-cells and antibodies. When the rats were given copper-enriched diets, their immune systems perked up.

No RDA has been set for copper, but 2 to 3 milligrams should be an adequate amount of this nutrient, says Tim Cramer, Ph.D., research professor in nutrition and immunity at the U.S. Department of Agriculture's Grand Forks Human Nutrition Center, North Dakota. Chicken, crabmeat, liver, cashews and whole grains are good copper sources.

OMEGA-3 FATTY ACIDS

You've just made a crisp salad with garden-fresh greens and vegetables. What's the healthiest way to top it off?

Before you drizzle on the salad dressing, how about adding some flaky chunks of pink salmon?

When it comes to keeping your immune system healthy, scientists are discovering that the oil in fatty fish like salmon, mackerel and herring may have big advantages over vegetable oil.

A Texas team of researchers headed by Michael Bennett, M.D., professor of pathology at the University of Texas Southwestern Medical Center in Dallas, compared the immune responses of mice fed three different diets. One diet contained vegetable fatty acids, another contained monounsaturated fatty acids (found in peanut and olive oils) and the third supplied fish oil. The mice were then injected with bacteria and cancer-causing chemicals, and their immune responses were measured.

The result? In the vegetable oil group, the T-cells were suppressed—they failed to respond against enemy substances. The monounsaturated fat group had less T-cell suppression. And the fish oil group had the least T-cell suppression of all.

Does this mean that if you douse your salads with safflower oil and eat cookies baked with vegetable oil, you're headed for trouble? "Not at all," Dr.

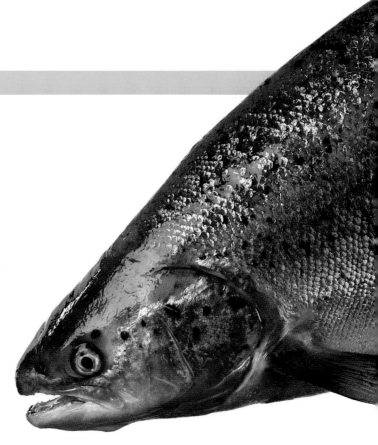

Bennett says. "What it does mean, though, is that if you are getting all of your fatty acids from vegetable oils and you run into, say, an influenza virus or even a carcinogen, your body may be less able to fight it."

The vegetable oil contains a type of fatty acid called omega-6, which contains arachidonic acid (AA). Researchers have discovered that in the body, AA produces E_2, which prevents the immune system from rallying against invaders.

Fish oil, on the other hand, is built of other kinds of polyunsaturated fatty acids, particularly eicosapentaenoic acid (EPA) and docosahexaenoic acid (DHA), which are designated omega-3. The omega-3 fatty acids do not make the prostaglandins.

Taming the Bad Fats

Fortunately, you can still go ahead and add that vegetable oil dressing to your tossed salad. It's possible, suggests Dr. Bennett, that by simply adding salmon and other fish to your diet, you could counteract any effects of vegetable oils.

Salmon is rich in omega-3, a kind of fatty acid that may give your immune system a helping hand.

"Some experts believe that if you add omega-3 fish oil to some omega-6 vegetable oils, it's the same as omega-3 alone," he says. In other words, omega-3 negates the destructive omega-6.

The theory is that in the cell membrane, omega-3 competes with omega-6 for the enzyme required to make prostaglandins. And omega-3 grabs it before omega-6 can do any harm.

One day you may be able to add specifically raised sea plants rich in omega-3 to your salads, Dr. Bennett ventures. Before that happens, though, you're more likely to see that your favorite vegetable oil has a new added ingredient: fish oil.

Soothing Inflammation

Fish oil may also become an important menu item for sufferers of certain autoimmune diseases, such as lupus.

In one study, mice genetically destined to get lupus (an inflammatory skin disease) were fed diets composed largely of either lard, corn oil or fish oil. Mice fed fish oil had less inflammation.

"Fish oil interferes with the prostaglandins, which are believed to cause the pain and inflammation in lupus," says researcher Thomas C. Clarkson, director of the Arteriosclerosis Research Center at Bowman Gray School of Medicine at Wake Forest University in Winston-Salem, North Carolina.

Similar results were found in human volun-

teers with rheumatoid arthritis, another autoimmune disease. Researchers at Albany Medical College gave 21 patients fish oil and 19 patients a look-alike placebo. After 14 weeks, they found that the fish oil group had less prostaglandin production and a decrease in the number of tender and swollen joints. What's more, the positive effects persisted four weeks after the fish oil supplementation was stopped.

Fish oil may not be a cure for this painful disease, according to one expert. But it appears to be a hopeful therapeutic approach, and for patients with rheumatoid arthritis, "there might be some merit in recommending dietary modification which involves increased fish consumption."

Picking the Best Fish

Just how much fish should you eat? "Two fish meals a week seems to reduce coronary problems," notes Dr. Clarkson. "But we don't know how much you need to keep the immune system healthy." With this in mind, here are some ways to get more omega-3 in your diet:

● Choose cold-water, deep-sea fish. Cold-water fish like sardines, salmon, tuna and mackerel feed on plankton, tiny sea plants rich in omega-3. And cold-water fish also have less saturated fat. (The more polyunsaturated the fat, the more liquid it remains at low temperature, enabling fish to survive in cold water.)

● Fresh is best. Frozen comes in second. Canned fish has the least amount of EPA. But you can get more omega-3 from canned tuna, for example, by choosing solid white albacore rather than chunk light. Buy the water-packed kind; you can drain off up to 25 percent of the fatty acids with the oil-packed kind.

● Not a fish fan? You can ask your doctor about fish oil supplements, keeping in mind that their ultimate safety has not been determined. Another point to consider: You would need to take more than five capsules of concentrated fish oil to give you as much EPA as a single 4-ounce serving of salmon provides.

OUTDOORS

Mountain lakes sparkling in the sunlight, thick belts of pine throwing fragrance into the air, dusty trails climbing to the snow line—that's the nature lover's view of the great outdoors.

And then, of course, there's the certified city-dweller's view: Streams packed full of microscopic bugs waiting to inflict pain and misery, forests crawling with little things that sting and big things that bite, and in all that vast expanse—no place to get out of the rain.

Who's right? Well, both. The outdoors can be beautiful, but it's often uncomfortable and dangerous, too, in ways that give your immune system a real workout.

James Wilkerson, M.D., author of *Medicine for Mountaineering,* is a nationally recognized authority on wilderness medicine. In his experience, the six threats to health listed below are those you're most likely to encounter outdoors.

DON'T DRINK THE WATER

The single biggest source of outdoor health problems is the water we drink when we're out there, Dr. Wilkerson says. And the most common result of bad water is diarrhea. But despite popular notions to the contrary, giardia—the generic name for mild diarrhea and fever caused by *Giardia lamblia* parasites—is not the chief villain.

"Everybody's scared of giardia, almost hysterical about it sometimes," Dr. Wilkerson says. "The Park Service will call a stream contaminated if they find a single organism in a hundred gallons of water. But in the vast majority of cases, other bugs are responsible for what the patient *thinks* is giardia—so much so that unless I see the organism actually cultured from a patient, I assume it's *not* giardia."

But if giardia wasn't to blame for that embarrassing episode on your last trip to Yosemite, then what was? Usually it's either a virus or bacteria, introduced into the body by drinking water contaminated with human waste, Dr. Wilkerson says.

Although antibiotics may be prescribed in special cases, most authorities recommend fluid replacement as the primary therapy until the diarrhea runs its course. So what to do if you want to avoid three days cloistered in the latrine?

It's simple, according to Dr. Wilkerson. Wash your hands before eating and disinfect your water. If you're within hailing distance of civilization, neither presents a problem. But getting clean water in the hinterlands can be difficult. Dr. Wil-

NEW WAYS TO MAKE YOUR WATER SAFE

Safe drinking water seems simple—until your first visit to a wilderness outfitter. Some say boil it. Some say filter it. And there are so many tablets to do it, you can't make up your mind.

James Wilkerson, M.D., recommends something called the Kahn-Visscher method. This technique relies on the powerful disinfection properties of crystalline iodine, which is available from chemical supply stores, along with a small, 30-milliliter glass bottle. To disinfect a quart of local water, the little bottle is filled with the crystalline iodine and shaken. After an hour, half of it is poured into the drinking water. Ten minutes later, the water is ready to drink.

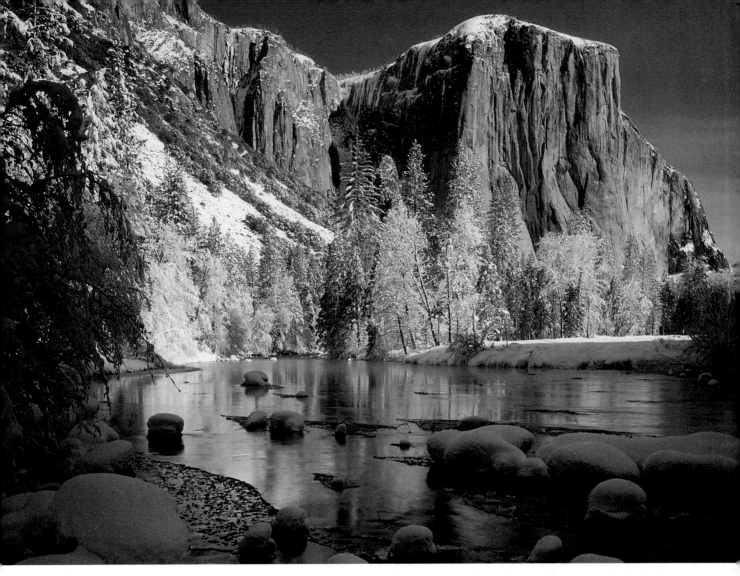

kerson's recommendation: Disinfect with iodine (see the box "New Ways to Make Your Water Safe" for details).

Other tactics all have their pitfalls. "Boiling is just too much of a hassle," Dr. Wilkerson says. "Most people won't do it. Filters work, but—no matter what the ads say—they don't eliminate virus particles. Chlorine binds with organic material, so getting the dose right can be a problem. And chlorine tablets degrade very quickly in the open air.

"But with iodine, all it takes is mixing the solution with your drinking water and then letting it sit for 10 minutes. *Everything* alive in that jug will die."

THE NOT-SO-GOOD EARTH

What's the second most common substance on earth? Earth—otherwise known as soil. And wherever you find soil, you'll find the bacteria responsible for tetanus, or lockjaw.

"It's endemic in the soil; there's just no way to avoid it," Dr. Wilkerson says. "The disease is usually

The sheer beauty of wilderness can obscure the risks. That crystalline clear water gorgeously aglitter in the mountain light may harbor *Giardia lamblia*—an organism that can cause mild dysentery.

introduced into the body through a cut or puncture, and it doesn't take much of a nick. There's not much you can do after it actually develops, and it's often fatal. The best thing you can do is keep your immunization up to date: Get a booster every ten years, or just before your trip."

Almost all Americans are inoculated against tetanus shortly after birth, but if you weren't, maybe two shots two months apart with a third six months later will firmly establish your immunity.

NERVOUS IN NEPAL

Wilderness enthusiasts who trek to the most remote and majestic corners of the globe risk an encounter with hepatitis B. This viral infection causes severe inflammation of the liver and can develop into

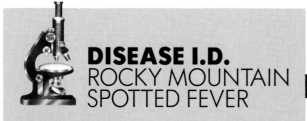

DISEASE I.D.
ROCKY MOUNTAIN SPOTTED FEVER

DESCRIPTION: Spotted fever is caused by bacteria (*Rickettsia rickettsii*) transmitted by tick bites. Initial symptoms include a rundown feeling and chills. The characteristic red rash—actually small hemorrhages in the skin—first appears on the wrists two to six days after the initial symptoms. Fever, headaches, generalized body pain, confusion and sensitivity to light follow.

INCIDENCE: Oddly enough, spotted fever isn't really found much in the Rocky Mountains anymore. "It's really an East Coast disease," says James Wilkerson, M.D. "You find an occasional case in the West, but Colorado tick fever is much more frequent there than Rocky Mountain spotted fever." The total U.S. cases in a recent year: 838.

MODE OF TRANSMISSION: Tick bites.

DEFENSE FACTORS: Make it hard for ticks to reach you with long-sleeved shirts, buttoned collars, and pants tucked into your boots. A hat doesn't hurt, and neither does staying out of the bushes—where you're most likely to pick up a tick. Use a repellent, and check yourself for ticks regularly (gasoline or fuel oil will make them drop off).

TREATMENT: If bitten, remove the tick and clean the bite site thoroughly. If fever develops or symptoms are severe, see a doctor. Dr. Wilkerson recommends tetracycline every 6 hours until the patient is free of fever for at least three days. Rest, aspirin and fluids complete the prescription.

RECOVERY TIME: If treated properly, symptoms should subside within 36 to 48 hours. Approximately 7 percent of all cases, however, are fatal.

chronic liver disease. It's also strongly linked to later liver cancer.

Hepatitis B is usually transmitted through contact with an infected person or something they've handled (often during meal preparation on the trail).

"You're more likely to get this traveling outside of the United States," Dr. Wilkerson says. "And for the most part, that's because sanitation is something that's just not understood in many parts of the world."

What to do? Since viral infections don't respond to antibiotics, treatment is chiefly a matter of prevention. The good news is that an effective vaccine is available that provides full immunity. Dr. Wilkerson recommends it for those planning a trip into undeveloped parts of the world.

WILD ABOUT WILDERNESS

Rabies is something we usually worry about dogs getting, but this infection is a threat to anyone who comes in contact with wild animals. Hikers and others who venture off the beaten track naturally run a bigger risk of the disease, which kills by causing severe inflammation of the brain.

"The virus is endemic in animal populations worldwide," says Dr. Wilkerson, "which means you can get it from a bite wherever you go, and it's uniformly fatal—if you get it, it kills you."

Here in the United States, rabies is most widespread among raccoons, bats, skunks and foxes. Squirrels and rabbits are almost never responsible for transmitting the disease, although they account for a large part of the bites reported each year. Excellent vaccination programs minimize the threat from dogs and cats, but abroad, it's a different story.

"Outside the United States, stay away from *any* animal, including pets. And if you do get bitten, get to an American embassy as fast as you can. The local vaccines are much more dangerous than the type we use, and the *only* place you'll find good rabies vaccine overseas is at the embassy."

Malaria isn't just the stuff of Indiana Jones thrillers, where the rugged hero swelters his way through a feverish attack wrapped in the arms of his

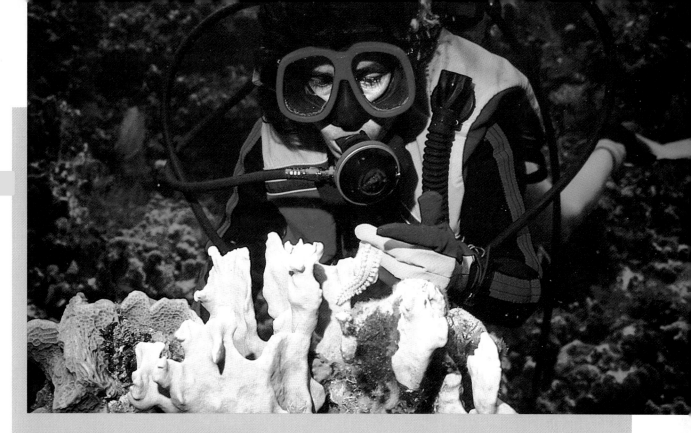

DEEP-SEA SCOUNDRELS

No, don't touch! If it were not for the protective underwater gloves she is wearing, sporting with this bristleworm perched on a crown of fire coral could mean double trouble for this scuba diver. Both are among the underwater menaces that can leave an unsuspecting diver with a wicked wound and possible infection. Though fragile and soft, the spines on the bristleworm are nee-

dle sharp. In an unfriendly encounter, the spines detach and become embedded in the skin, causing pain similar to a fiberglass cut. To get the spines out, experts recommend using Scotch tape, although there is little you can do for the pain. A brush with fire coral can leave painful red welts on the skin that can last a long time. An application of meat tenderizer will help get the fire out.

gorgeous native sweetheart. In some parts of the world, it's an everyday possibility for anyone who ventures outdoors.

Insect repellent and long-sleeved shirts can cut your risk in high-danger areas like Central America. But malaria is still one of the world's most prevalent diseases, with millions of people infected worldwide, including more than 1,000 reported cases in the southeastern United States in a recent year.

Caused by a mosquito-borne parasite that literally eats your red blood cells, malaria typically produces chills, fever, muscle aches and the notorious cold sweats. On the positive side, in many instances malaria can be effectively prevented with drugs.

A SHOCKING REACTION

Even a bug that isn't carrying a hostile organism hungry for human meat can cause problems. According to Dr. Wilkerson, allergic reactions to insect

stings are another major outdoor health threat.

"For most of us, stings aren't a problem," Dr. Wilkerson says. "But there's a significant minority of people at risk of anaphylactic shock—massive allergic reaction to a sting or bite that can cause death. The problem here is that the patient can die within 5 minutes without appropriate treatment."

Fortunately, you don't have to eliminate the outdoors from your recreational agenda even if you are allergic to bug bites. "Epinephrine—adrenaline—is essential and effective treatment for anaphylactic shock, and it's available now in injectors you can use with one hand," says Dr. Wilkerson. "You just punch your thigh with the device and it delivers a measured dose into the muscle."

If you're sensitive, make the injectors part of your prehike packing. And pack several, Dr. Wilkerson advises, since it may take repeated injections to control your allergic reaction.

PETS

Zoonoses: If the authors of "Dick and Jane" primers had tried to explain the term to you back in elementary school, their lesson might have read something like this:

> Look, Jane, look.
> Spot is sick.
> Cough, Spot, cough.
> Play with Spot.
> Catch Spot's germs.
> Germs, germs, germs.

Zoonoses, or zoonotic diseases, are infections you can catch from animals. There are more than 30 such diseases, and you don't have to own an exotic South American bird or a Gila monster to be at risk. In many cases, the culprits are Spot, Fluffy or one of the other 100 million or more cats and dogs Americans keep as pets.

Most zoonoses aren't exactly everyday household words. Take toxoplasmosis, for instance, a cat-borne parasite that's dangerous for pregnant women (see the box "Vaccine on the Horizon for Toxoplasmosis"). But "cat scratch fever," transmitted by—what else?—cat scratches, may sound more familiar. Even worse than scratches are bites, which carry the deadly potential of transmitting rabies (see "Disease I.D.: Rabies" on page 109). Every year, about a half million Americans (mostly children) have a chunk taken out of them by animals.

Considering the amount of time Dick and Jane spend with Spot and Fluffy, however, the chances of getting illnesses from a pet are actually pretty slight. And for the most part, these illnesses can be prevented.

CLEAN UP YOUR ACT

"Ninety percent of prevention is a matter of cleanliness," says Jill Frucci, D.V.M., editor of the *Journal of the American Animal Hospital Association*. "If you're normally clean, you're not going to have a problem."

Pucker up for your pet? Go right ahead. You're no more likely to get an infectious disease from kissing a dog than from kissing a person.

You should pay special attention to the following factors.

Litter box and living quarters. Change your cat's litter every week or so, says Dr. Frucci. Between times, remove stools, which carry bacteria, worms and assorted parasites. Use a scooper or toilet paper and dispose of the offending substance promptly.

Apply the same standards of cleanliness to Fluffy's basket or Spot's doghouse. If you use a sponge to clean up any animal mess, just rinsing it out won't kill the germs. Throw it away. And be sure to wash your hands afterward.

Your pet. Some breeds of dogs need a bath on a regular basis, others don't. If Spot counts himself among the dirty dogs, start scrubbing. Cats generally clean themselves, and it's a good thing, too: Water enthusiasts they are not. "I never give my cat a bath," says Dr. Frucci. She suggests an occasional cleanup with a fresh towel and a combing instead.

If you share sleeping quarters with your pet, you certainly don't want Spot's dirt or Fluffy's fleas in your bed. "I don't care where you live, whether it's Alaska or Florida, you're going to face some kind of parasite problem," says Dr. Frucci. Although fleas and mites find pets a lot tastier than people, they will take an occasional bite out of you. These can leave their mark in serious infections like Kawasaki disease, which can damage your heart. Declare war on fleas, using collars, powders, sprays, a flea comb, professional dip or whatever else works.

Your kids. Children are more susceptible to zoonoses because "they're shorter, closer to the ground," says Dr. Frucci. "They're always putting the cat's tail in their mouths, licking the dog's ears. It's the nature of kids." Make sure your kids aren't digging trenches in your cat's litter box or eating lunch in the doghouse.

BACK OFF FROM BITES

When it comes to bites and scratches, caution is the best medicine.

"Don't put yourself in a compromising situation," says Dr. Frucci. "If your dog is growling, back off.

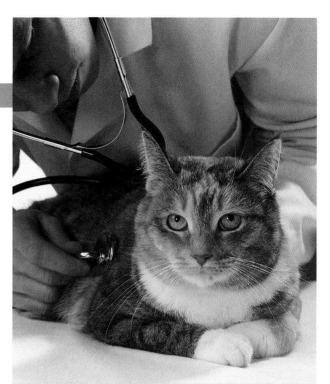

VACCINE ON THE HORIZON FOR TOXOPLASMOSIS

It occurs very rarely, but when it does, the effects can be heartbreaking. Toxoplasmosis, a parasitic disease of cats transmitted to people by cat feces, can cause birth defects when pregnant women are infected. About 3,000 infants born each year suffer mental retardation or vision problems as a result. There is no known cure for toxoplasmosis.

But there's good news on the horizon. Researchers are developing a vaccine that would prevent cats from getting toxoplasmosis in the first place. The vaccine gives the cat a mutant strain of the parasite, which fools the animal's system into becoming immune to the real thing.

The beauty of the vaccine is that cats rather than people will be immunized, says researcher Elmer Pfefferkorn, Ph.D., professor and chairman of microbiology at Dartmouth Medical School. Thus, the parasite will be blocked before it can be transmitted. Dr. Pfefferkorn says the vaccine will not be commercially available until the 1990s. Meanwhile, pregnant women should avoid contact with litter boxes.

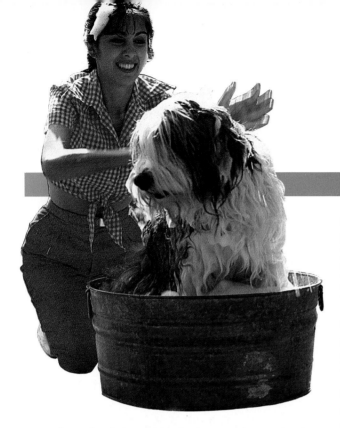

Your dog's bath is an ideal opportunity to check for fleas and mites, which can cause allergies and carry disease.

Don't try to pull a bone out of his mouth. And don't ever jump into the middle of a dog or cat fight."

Last, a note about zoonoses in reverse: Medical evidence suggests that *you* could be making your pet sick. "I've seen lots of people who say, 'I had the flu last week and now my dog is sick,'" says Dr. Frucci. So if you're ill, what does the doctor prescribe to help you keep your germs to yourself? "Simple," she says. "Stop coughing and hacking in Fluffy's face."

THE HEALTHY DOG

Your dog is susceptible to hundreds of diseases, many of them very painful, some fatal. Take canine distemper, for instance, a highly contagious virus transmitted from one dog to another through the air. Or canine parvovirus, which infected dogs in a nationwide epidemic in the 1970s. Or rabies.

These and other deadly diseases are often not treatable once Spot starts showing symptoms. But with a little dogged determination, you can protect him.

Vaccinations, the first line of defense. For starters, see that your dog is vaccinated early and annually, says Amy Marder, V.M.D., clinical assistant professor at Tufts University School of Veterinary Medicine. Not only can Spot catch diseases from animals outside or pet pals at home, he can also contract viruses floating by through the air or carried on your clothes and shoes. Take your puppy for his first vaccination when he's eight weeks old. Follow up with booster shots as recommended by your veterinarian.

Good nutrition. When it comes to your dog's ability to resist disease, "proper nutrition is imperative," says Peter Jezyk, V.M.D., professor of medicine and medical genetics at the University of Pennsylvania Veterinary School. "Studies show that malnourished animals have very poor immune responses, whereas a well-balanced diet maintains a healthy immune system."

How do you choose from the zillions of dog food brands and flavors barking for your attention in the pet food aisle? Michael Garvey, D.V.M., chairman of the Department of Medicine at the Animal Medical Center in New York and coauthor of *The Complete Book of Dog Health,* offers this general rule: "For your average dog, one who is not under any excess physical or emotional stress, just about any nutritionally balanced, name-brand dog food will be fine." Your puppy, however, will require specially formulated food to avoid harmful nutritional deficiencies.

Good food and lots of it is especially important when Spot is sick. "A dog with a severe infection could need five times as many calories as usual to maintain his immune system responses," says Dr. Jezyk.

Fight fat. On the other hand, don't let Spot get fat. You may think he looks awfully cute bouncing around in an impersonation of a four-legged beach ball, but he'll be a lot more resistant to disease if he is at normal weight.

"Obesity lowers resistance," says Dr. Jezyk. "The immune system in general doesn't function as well in animals that are fat."

Keeping an eye on the scale is especially important when Spot is still a little tyke. Studies show that animals that are kept on the lean side as they're growing up have a stronger immune system and do better throughout life.

As many as 40 percent of dogs in the United States are overweight, according to the American Animal Hospital Association. Feel for Spot's ribs along the sides of his body. If he doesn't seem to have any, it's time for a doggy diet.

Resisting your desire to treat Spot to a helping of your sumptuous supper can keep his weight down, too. So can keeping him out of the garbage, which also protects him from the fast-breeding bacteria that flourish there. Since scavenging comes naturally to Spot's species—and to cats, too, by the way—feeding him a well-balanced diet at home won't necessarily discourage him. Your best bet is to hound him not to crash anyone's trash in the first place.

Physical fitness. Unlike humans, exercise in a dog isn't directly linked to his immune power. At least no studies thus far show a connection, says Dr. Jezyk. However, Spot's cardiovascular system is strengthened by exercise and hence will be better able to deliver disease-fighting blood cells to injured tissues.

Home health check. Play doctor with Spot during his bath time or brushing. It's an ideal opportunity to give him an overall health check. Feel him all over, looking for lumps, sores and anything else unusual. And check for fleas, ticks and other parasites, which can transmit anything from tapeworm to bubonic plague. Fleas can also cause a painful skin reaction called flea allergic dermatitis. Both dogs and cats are especially likely to be allergic if they were exposed to lots of fleas when they were young.

Home away from home. On occasion, you may need to put Spot in a kennel for a couple of days while you're away. This can expose him to diseases his immune system has never seen before. Make sure you get him vaccinated seven to ten days in advance of the kennel stay to give him a chance to build up immunity, says Dr. Jezyk.

Visit the vet. An annual visit to your veterinarian will include Spot's booster shots and tests to detect problems early. See your vet, too, if your dog displays a change in habits, personality or activity level—the most common signs of illness.

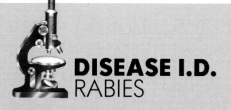

DISEASE I.D.
RABIES

DESCRIPTION: A fatal viral disease in dogs, cats and other warm-blooded animals. Symptoms, which result from inflammation of the brain, begin with personality changes in which the pet behaves in uncharacteristic ways. These are followed by one of two forms of the disease: the paralytic form, in which the swallowing muscles of the throat are paralyzed and the animal drools, coughs or paws at its mouth, or the "mad dog" type in which the animal becomes frenzied and vicious and attacks all animals and people in its path. Contrary to popular belief, foaming at the mouth is not a common symptom.

INCIDENCE: In 1986, rabies was reported in 94 dogs and 166 cats in the United States. Nearly twice as many cases were recorded in 1981—an unusually high number. Overall, the number of rabid dogs and cats has decreased in the past decade.

MODE OF TRANSMISSION: Because the rabies virus is present in saliva, infection is passed primarily through a bite from an infected animal. Bats, foxes, raccoons and other warm-blooded wild animals (though not rodents like rats, mice and squirrels) can be carriers. Humans can contract it, too.

DEFENSE FACTORS: Vaccinations are essential for all dogs and cats, beginning when they are several weeks old and continuing annually. To protect yourself and your animal, do not get near any potentially rabid animal. If you suspect your pet has been bitten by any wild animal, see your vet immediately. Do not wait for symptoms; they can take several weeks to develop.

TREATMENT: There is no effective treatment for the disease in animals.

RECOVERY TIME: No recovery known.

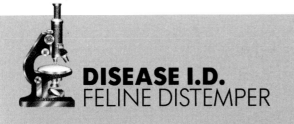

DISEASE I.D.
FELINE DISTEMPER

DESCRIPTION: A serious and often fatal viral disease in cats (especially kittens). Also known as feline panleukopenia, early symptoms include loss of appetite, vomiting and depression. The virus damages the digestive tract and destroys the immune system's disease-fighting white blood cells, which results in a massive infection throughout the bloodstream. It can come on very suddenly and severely without apparent warning.

INCIDENCE: Frequent among unvaccinated cats and especially widespread among the feral cat population (those living in the wild).

MODES OF TRANSMISSION: Most cats are exposed to this highly contagious virus sometime during their lives. It is spread by direct contact with an infected cat or his secretions, through the air or by exposure to contaminated litter boxes or food pans. Resistant to ordinary household disinfectants, the virus can live for at least a year in carpets, cracks and furnishings.

DEFENSE FACTORS: Vaccination is the primary form of prevention and is essential whether your cat lives indoors or is allowed outside. See your veterinarian for your kitten's first shot when he is about eight weeks old. Your adult cat should receive a booster shot every year. To disinfect infected household areas, use a diluted chlorine bleach solution.

TREATMENT: The earlier you notice the symptoms and get your cat to a veterinarian, the better, as death may come quickly. While the virus itself cannot be combated, the dangerous symptoms can. Intensive treatment consists of intravenous fluids, supplemental nutrition, antibiotics and, in some cases, blood transfusions.

RECOVERY TIME: Can take weeks while the virus runs its course.

THE HEALTHY CAT

Whoever said that the cat has nine lives neglected to inform Fluffy's immune system. Cats are susceptible to a great many diseases, and some of the most common ones are deadly, says Tufts University's Dr. Marder. Feline urologic syndrome, or FUS, for example, is a serious urinary tract problem that strikes one out of ten cats. And feline leukemia acts like AIDS does in human beings, suppressing the immune system and leaving its victim prone to diseases like respiratory infections and cancer.

But with proper care there's lots of hope for making Fluffy's one life a long one.

Vaccinations. Protect your cat against feline leukemia, deadly distemper (see the accompanying box), rabies and an assortment of viruses with a simple shot. Well, a few simple shots. When your kitten is about eight weeks old, see your veterinarian for the first of a series of vaccinations, followed by a booster shot every year, says Dr. Marder. And get her vaccinated whether she's an indoor or outdoor cat to protect her against infections that travel via clothes or through the air.

Disease-resistant diet. Fluffy may love tuna straight from the can, but her immunity to disease will be less of a fishy business with proper nutrition. Name-brand cat foods labeled "nutritionally balanced" are just what she needs. If Fluffy's still a kitten, look for foods specially balanced for her growing needs.

Researchers believe you might be able to keep Fluffy from a bout with FUS by feeding her foods low in ash. This is especially important if Fluffy is actually Freddy; your male cat can develop serious urethral blockage from the disease. Compare labels on cans to make your selections.

As with Spot, Fluffy's immune system will be stronger if she stays slim. One way to keep her weight down, especially if she's an indoor cat, is to stock up on cat toys and play with her. Be careful, though, not to let her play with string, yarn and other potentially dangerous objects. Swallowing something sharp could perforate her intestines and lead to peritonitis, a very serious challenge to the immune system.

A good licking. Cats do a fine job of cleaning themselves, but they need your occasional assistance. Combating fleas, for instance, requires lots of environmental prevention and maybe even—if you dare try it—a bath. And remember that whatever substances cats get on their fur, they'll lick off, whether it's motor oil or disease-infected feces deposited in your driveway by other animals. At the very least, wipe off suspicious substances with a damp towel.

The indoor/outdoor dilemma. The decision whether to keep Fluffy indoors or let her roam free in the great outdoors can be a tough one. Outdoor cats enjoy more freedom and aren't frustrated by confinement, says Dr. Marder. The indoor cat, however, is a lot less likely to come in contact with contagious diseases or to contract infection from scavenging through your neighbors' garbage cans.

Stress management. As with Spot, make sure Fluffy is vaccinated well in advance of her stay at a kennel. Not only can she catch a bug from a fellow kennel guest, but the very stress of changing environments can make her sick.

"Stress can lower immunity in animals. There's no question about that," says Dr. Jezyk. "If you take a cat to a veterinary office for a blood sample, you can see indicators of stress in the blood—high glucose levels, changes in the white blood cell count—in just a few minutes."

Visit the vet. Get Fluffy to the veterinarian every year for booster shots and a checkup. And consult the doctor if your cat displays the common signs of illness: a change in habits, personality or appetite.

Remember, too, that doing your part to keep Fluffy and Spot healthy is a lifelong process. Don't make the mistake of growing lax as your pets grow older, says Dr. Jezyk. The fact is, your pets have weakened immune responses overall as they age. They're also more likely to develop something called immune-mediated diseases, which are related to abnormalities in the immune system.

So keep Spot and Fluffy on a balanced diet every day, and get them to the doctor regularly for a checkup and updated vaccinations. They will reward you with happy, healthy companionship for many more years to come.

Extra protection for your outdoor cat includes neutering and a flea collar. Vaccinate him, too, of course, but *don't* declaw him.

PLAGUE

nter through the portal of time to Paris, 1348. A terrible epidemic of bubonic plague is sweeping over Europe, and well beyond. Each day, nearly 800 are dying in the French capital alone. Within a year, half of Paris, two-thirds of Venice and as much as four-fifths of Florence will be gone. Vienna, Hamburg and Avignon will be devastated. In fact, few cities will be spared.

If we stay through this dark age until the end of the century, we'll see between a quarter and a third—some estimates say as much as half—of all Europe fall to the epidemic that will one day be known as the Black Death. Among all the outbreaks of all the diseases of history, it will have no peer.

This epidemic of epidemics made "plague" a household word. But, like other once-specific names that have worked their way into our language as generic descriptions, the word *plague* has undergone a transformation. It's hardly used anymore to signify the specific disease of bubonic plague, but instead now stands for any social ill, like drug abuse or, more often, any epidemic disease. We speak often, for instance, of the AIDS *plague*.

Concern over AIDS, and speculation as to how far it can spread, has sparked interest in the epidemics of yesteryear. And of all yesteryear's epidemics, the horrible Black Death has been the most extensively studied and is therefore the best known.

What do we know about it? We know bubonic plague is still very much alive, however rare. There

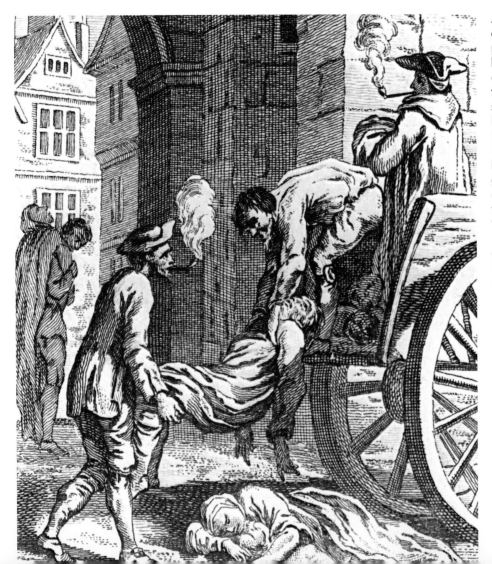

Although the largest epidemic of bubonic plague occurred in the late 1340s, periodic outbreaks hit Europe throughout the next several centuries. The horror of such an outbreak in 17th-century England is depicted in this 19th-century engraving. The puffing of pipes was believed to keep away the "bad air," thought by many to cause the disease. At the very least, the aromatic smoke probably helped to mask the unpleasant smell of death.

were 12 cases in the United States in one recent year. Can it reach epidemic proportions again? How does a disease like plague so devastate one generation, die out, then rear its ugly head to torture some far-distant generation? What do AIDS and other modern-day plagues have in common with the Black Death? What role does the immune system play in warding off or inviting epidemic diseases?

WHAT EPIDEMICS ARE MADE OF

"The rise and decline of epidemics is the product of an extremely complicated ecology," says Guenter Risse, M.D., Ph.D., chairman of the Department of History of Health Sciences at the University of California at San Francisco. In other words, it's hard to pin the rap for an epidemic on any one thing.

Changes in climate; the movement of human populations; the migration of rats, fleas, mosquitoes and ticks; the decline or improvement of public sanitation; the natural mutation of viruses and bacteria; varying human population densities, social customs and housing conditions; and the availability of vaccines and antibiotics—all have interacted through the years to give us our historical log of epidemics.

Certainly a large factor is immunity. Individuals, once exposed to an invading organism, develop antibodies to that organism and so become less susceptible to its next uninvited visit. So, too, entire populations may develop (or lack) immunity.

Thanks to such a discrepancy among populations, fewer than 600 Spanish soldiers conquered the entire Aztec empire simply by carrying to the New World all of the common childhood diseases of the Old World. Measles and smallpox proved powerful ammunition in a land devoid of antibodies. The ensuing and unrelenting epidemics among the native Mexicans reduced their numbers from roughly 30 million in the 1520s, when the Spaniards arrived, to a mere 1.6 million by the 1620s!

Immunity is influenced not only by heredity and previous exposure to harmful organisms but by lifestyle as well. Diet plays a particularly significant

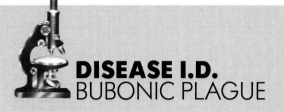

DISEASE I.D.
BUBONIC PLAGUE

DESCRIPTION: The disease takes its name from the buboes—swellings in the lymph nodes of the groin, armpit or neck—that victims typically develop. Other symptoms include chills, fever, nausea, stomach cramps and rapid pulse. In later stages, the blood may coagulate under the skin, resulting in a blackening of the body, beginning with fingers, toes and nose. Without treatment, this bacterial infection is often fatal.

INCIDENCE: Once the scourge of humanity, plague has largely been brought under control. There were 12 isolated cases in the western United States in one recent year.

MODES OF TRANSMISSION: Humans usually contract the disease by flea bite. The bacteria-carrying fleas are most commonly found living off the backs of rodents—primarily rats and squirrels. Direct contact with an infected animal can also lead to trouble.

DEFENSE FACTORS: If you live in or visit a high-risk area—particularly New Mexico, Arizona, California, Colorado, or Utah—avoid wild rodents and their fleas. Keep your pets flea-free. Do not handle sick or dead wild animals.

TREATMENT: Should you suspect plague, see a physician immediately. Hospitalization and rapid treatment with antibiotics will increase your chance of survival from slim to excellent.

RECOVERY TIME: If diagnosed and treated in its early stages, the disease can be knocked out in one to two weeks.

role. A malnourished child living in the foothills of Guatemala could easily die of measles, says Dr. Risse. In contrast, a well-fed child in New York will typically shake the disease in a matter of days. So, hungry countries are more prone to epidemics than well-fed ones. Right?

Well, yes and no. Recent studies are drawing all kinds of parallels between good nutrition and strong immunity. Some findings, however, are raising sticky questions, says Dr. Risse. For example, sub-Saharan Africans suffering from severe malnourishment remain astonishingly free of many epidemics raging around them, "only to show symptoms of disease when they begin to get fed again," says Dr. Risse. One explanation may be that the organisms invading the body of a starved person can't get enough nutrients themselves to grow and create havoc.

To see how immunity and the other factors mentioned earlier interact, let's again turn to the epidemic disease about which we know the most—the Black Death.

THE HISTORY OF PLAGUE

What bubonic plague was, or what caused it, wasn't understood until the late 19th century when Robert Koch and Louis Pasteur first began to make the connection between microorganisms and disease. The *Yersinia pestis* bacterium was finally identified as the villain, clearing the name of all that had been blamed for the plague since ancient times, including bad air, loose living, heretics and, well, "you name it," says John Parascandola, Ph.D., chief of the History Division at the National Library of Medicine.

Plague was known during biblical times, having reportedly infected the Philistines about 1320 B.C. The first recorded intercontinental epidemic was the bubonic plague outbreak of the 6th century, the so-called Plague of Justinian, which blanketed North Africa, the Middle East and southern Europe.

But, prior to the Black Death, "our model for all epidemics," says Dr. Parascandola, bubonic plague was relatively unknown, at least in Europe, for centuries. How then could it have burst out in late 1347 with such venom as to strike down as many as 25 to 50 million people in the next three years? "The conditions," says Dr. Parascandola, "were ripe."

The social and biological conditions of the time forged the perfect cauldron in which bacteria, fleas, rodents and humans could all combine to form an infectious brew. The plague bacteria were carried by fleas, which were carried by rats, which, in the squalor of the age, often lived under the same roofs with humans.

Scientists think these rats came to Europe by hitching rides in the wagons of Crusaders returning from the Holy Land. Incessant wars and political instability had rendered the continent poor, its people hungry and its new cities crowded and filthy. As the plague began to take hold, the enormous number of deaths resulted in more fallow fields and more unkempt streets than before. With more poverty, more filth, more famine and more of all the things that rats so cherish, they multiplied. Along with the fleas and bacteria.

Plague spread from town to town with the newly created merchant class, the traveling salesmen. Not only did the peddlers carry rats in their wagons and goods, but the sick often developed a pneumonic phase of the disease, when they themselves could become carriers, and spread the scourge with their violent sneezes.

More men than women died of plague. One theory holds that since men ventured from home more often than women, they were more likely to pick up the disease. But another theory holds accountable the plague bacteria's taste for iron. It is presumed that nearly all women during the Middle Ages were iron deficient, just as many women are today. Men, who ate more food and needed less of the nutrient, had plenty for the bacteria to thrive on.

And the bacteria thrived. By 1350, however, plague passed from most of the European continent. It reappeared in spurts throughout the next 350 years, to peter out almost entirely by the end of the 1600s. Why?

Surely, the disease's disappearance had little to

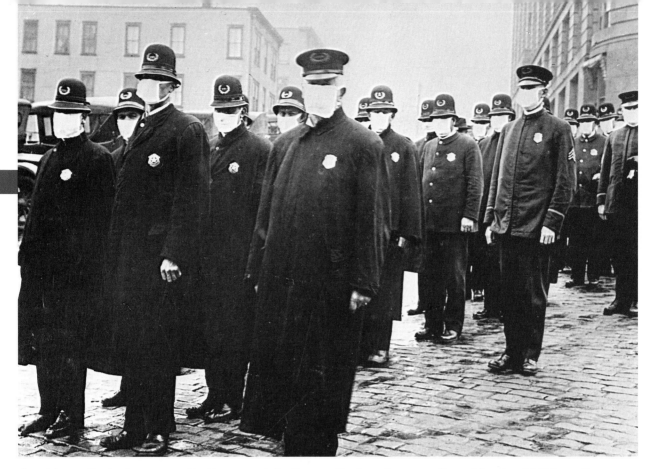

During the great flu epidemic of 1918, policemen did more than wear masks—in some cities they arrested people who didn't. Pictured here are some of Seattle's finest.

do with medical science, says Dr. Parascandola. During the Black Death, doctors often wore long-beaked masks to scare away lurking demons. They prescribed a number of remedies similarly lacking in scientific value. Plague victims were treated with bloodletting, with laxatives and enemas and with pills of crushed stag's horn. As preventives, people were urged to eat lentils, suck sour plums, drink onion juice and stop having sex.

Obviously, other factors were more influential. Public sanitation improved. Quarantines were ordered (although germs weren't understood, it was observed that plague sometimes passed from person to person). In addition, it's theorized that rats may have roamed less, and so were less apt to pick up infected fleas from other rats.

Why the Black Death virtually vanished will probably never be fully known. What remains today is the mystery, the tales of woe and the imprecise records. We are left with remnants of the disease itself.

PLAGUE THROUGH THE MODERN DAY

In a case that has become somewhat famous, on March 6, 1900, the body of a Chinese man was removed from the basement of the Globe Hotel in San Francisco. An autopsy revealed plague. The dead man's house and the undertaker's shop were sprayed. But it was too late. Plague had finally come to America, most likely in the same manner it had arrived in Europe six centuries earlier: with travelers from afar.

Fear and ignorance led to panic. City authorities placed a cordon around 12 blocks of Chinatown; 35,000 people were quarantined. All Asiatics were barred from travel. Strict laws governed the city. All to little avail. The ensuing San Francisco epidemic killed 118. Later epidemics would occur in San Francisco and Seattle (1907), New Orleans (1912) and Los Angeles (1924). Since the Los Angeles epidemic, the last America would experience, plague cases have cropped up only in isolated incidents.

What happens to a disease like plague when it's not laying waste to nations? Where does it go? It lives on in the animal kingdom. Plague in the United States today survives in rural and suburban rodents—squirrels, rabbits and prairie dogs, and their fleas. The disease occasionally may be passed to or through other wildlife and even domestic cats and dogs, says Allan Barnes, Ph.D., chief of the federal Centers for Disease Control (CDC) plague branch in picturesque

Fort Collins, Colorado.

Most human cases result from flea bites, although sometimes there is direct contact with an infected animal. The main weapon we have against bubonic plague today in the United States, says Dr. Barnes, is the control of wild rodents and fleas. He also emphasizes the need for the education of inhabitants and physicians in high-risk areas.

Where are the high-risk areas? "Anything west of Dallas, but particularly northern central New Mexico, followed by Arizona, California, Colorado and Utah," says Thomas Quan, Ph.D., a microbiologist at the CDC plague lab who is currently working to develop new methods for rapid diagnosis of the disease. Because plague is now treatable with antibiotics, the few deaths that do occur are the result of patients not seeking medical care quickly enough or of physicians not recognizing the disease. "Everyone thinks it's a disease of antiquity, even

doctors," says Dr. Quan. This "disease of antiquity" infected roughly 200 Americans just in the last decade, of which better than 80 percent survived, he says.

Antibiotic treatment aside, the best measure is prevention of the disease in the first place. Should you live in or visit a high-risk area, Dr. Quan and his colleagues suggest you take the following precautions:

• Avoid contact with squirrels, rabbits and other wild rodents.

• Do not camp anywhere near such animals' burrows (remember that fleas are champion jumpers).

• Keep your pets free of fleas. It's best to keep them inside as much as possible. Don't take them on camping trips.

• Do not touch any sick or dead animal. Hunters should wear rubber gloves when dressing or skinning game.

• If you experience any of the signs of plague—

HOW PLAGUE IS SPREAD

During the Black Death of the 1300s, most victims contracted plague from infected fleas springing off the backs of black rats. Today, as illustrated at right, infected fleas jumping off rural rodents, and sometimes domestic animals, are the main problem. Humans may also contract plague through direct contact with rodents or with rodent-eating cats.

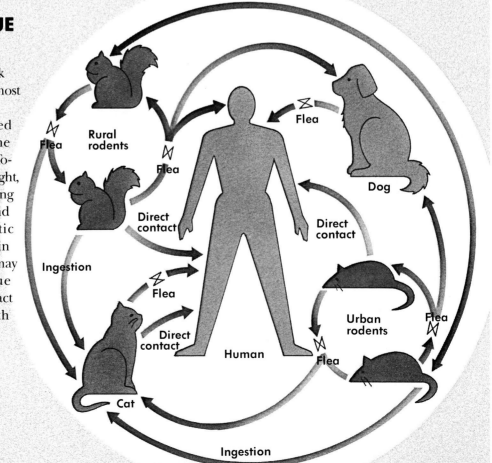

Flea

Rural rodents

Flea

Flea

Direct contact

Ingestion

Flea

Direct contact

Cat

Ingestion

Human

Flea

Dog

Direct contact

Urban rodents

Flea

Flea

swelling, chills, fever, cramps and rapid pulse—see a doctor. Fast. The disease is only curable if treated quickly.

Outside of the American West, plague today is still a problem in Madagascar, Burma, Vietnam, Brazil, Ecuador, Peru, Bolivia and South Africa.

PLAGUE'S COUSINS

Most epidemics of the late 20th century, at least in economically developed countries, involved chronic diseases—such as heart disease and cancer—rather than infectious diseases. AIDS is a notable exception. So is flu. In other parts of the world, where public sanitation is poor and rodents and insects run rampant, some of history's great infectious killers still take their toll: cholera, typhoid, typhus, yellow fever.

Are conditions now ripe for AIDS to spread wild, or for other infectious diseases to take hold? As for AIDS, Dr. Barnes says this disease, which is usually sexually transmitted, "has nothing to do with bubonic plague except that they both kill people." In other words, because AIDS is not transmitted by casual contact or by animals, it is unlikely that it will rip through 20th-century America the way the Black Death spread through 14th-century Europe. That's *not* to say AIDS isn't a growing problem—it is.

Is AIDS our biggest worry? Modern science, some fear, has the ability to unleash infectious epidemics that could make the Black Death seem as dangerous as acne. "The most dangerous bacteria and viruses known to mankind—as well as some that have never existed before—are currently being made in military laboratories, where gene-splicing technologies are being perfected under defense department contracts with universities, corporations and government," says popular author and lecturer Jeremy Rifkin. He says the possibility that these deadly organisms will accidentally escape from the laboratory and be unleashed on a public with limited or no immunity is all too real.

Freak accidents or germ warfare aside, epidemics of one form or another will follow us into the future. We hope that bubonic plague, cholera and

THE WAGES OF SIN

"AIDS is a lethal judgment of God on the sin of homosexuality," said evangelist Jerry Falwell.

Stern words. But Reverend Falwell is not alone these days in attributing the world's most recent epidemic to sin. In fact, historians say, such accusations are as common and as old as disease itself.

"We've always looked for scapegoats to explain what we don't understand," says John Parascandola, Ph.D. "Whenever a new disease arises, with yet no scientific explanation, it's easy to look for other explanations."

So when French soldiers of the 1400s entered Naples and an outbreak of syphilis followed, it was natural, says Dr. Parascandola, for both the French and the Neopolitans to blame the disease on the ungodly ways of the other. The affliction for years was referred to as either the "Neopolitan" or the "French" disease—depending, of course, on who was talking.

During the Black Death, when no one knew that rats and fleas were to blame for bubonic plague, the culprits often became Jews and lepers (who were said to join forces at night to poison the wells). Although they certainly suffered from the disease as much as any group, Jews throughout Europe were burned at the stake.

As for the Reverend Falwell's denunciation of homosexuals, it is the past repeating itself: "Very typical," says Guenter Risse, M.D., Ph.D. "There is perhaps a certain reassurance in knowing that this is not the first time this has happened, nor is it likely to be the last."

yellow fever will eventually go the way of smallpox, into total oblivion. But AIDS is probably here to stay, for a while at least. And who can predict when another new malady like Legionnaires' disease will appear? Or when the common flu virus will mutate into something more dangerous, as it has already done several times in the last century?

To think we will ever live in a world totally devoid of disease is "preposterous," says Dr. Risse. All the same, it's clear to see that we've come a long way since the Black Death in learning to keep diseases under control.

REGIONAL INFECTIONS

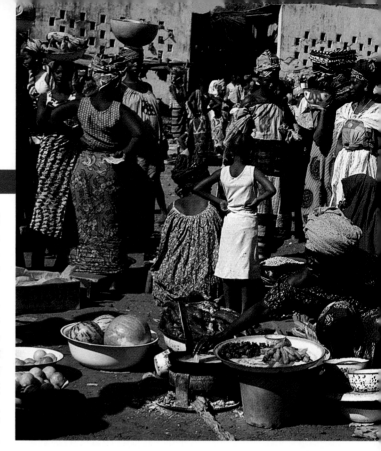

Y ou may enjoy sipping margaritas under a broiling Caribbean sun. Your neighbor is more the ski Colorado type. You may like lots of foliage around you, lush and green. A friend of yours prefers the throbbing city.

Bacteria, viruses and parasites are the same way.

Generally speaking, most infectious agents like their surroundings warm, moist and a tad on the grimy side. But this still leaves a lot of room for individual tastes. Some organisms, such as the omnipresent Salmonella, will set up house just about anywhere. Others, like the recently discovered Lassa virus, found only in certain rat-plagued areas of sub-Saharan Africa, are extremely fussy about where they'll call home.

On these pages, we take a glimpse at a few of the world's most persnickety little critters and the regional infections they're known to cause. None of the following are as common as malaria or yellow fever—ailments that have flared up over continents and wide populations. And certainly, says John Moran, M.D., medical adviser to the Peace Corps, the following infections are nothing for most Americans, even traveling Americans, to worry too much about.

Nevertheless, they can be devastating to local populations. They are also a bit bizarre. And be forewarned, these afflictions can be a little revolting, as is the case with the first few we'll describe.

SOUTHERN SCOURGES

You might suspect that the climates of the southern countries would be the perfect environment for some unusual diseases, and you are right. Here's a sampling of what the residents of some of those areas have to watch out for.

Elephantiasis. This affliction, which is found only in the hottest and steamiest areas of Africa, Asia and South America, is possibly the most curious disease in the world. The criminal element here is the tiny Wuchereria worm, which finds its way under the skin via certain tropical blood-sucking flies and mosquitoes. If the infection is not detected and treated early, its victims—as the name of the disease implies—develop grotesque, elephantlike, nearly elephant-*size* body parts. The affliction is extraordinarily hideous because it often affects the legs and scrotum, making walking impossible. Once elephantiasis has set in, it has no known cure, although chemotherapy treatments and draining of the infected appendages can keep the symptoms somewhat under control.

African sleeping sickness. This disease is also transmitted by flies—the infamous tsetse flies of darkest Africa. They carry not parasitic worms but wiggly, string-bean-shaped microorganisms called Trypanosomes. Usually, victims discover a painful red chancre within a few days after being bitten. Within several weeks, a high fever typically develops. This is only the beginning of their troubles. The infected person may later experience muscular rigidity, tremors and—most notably—extreme fatigue. Eventually, untreated victims, although feeling euphoric, grow comatose and, invariably, die. If, however, the proper medications are given before the final stages set in, the condition can be reversed.

Chagas disease. Found across the Atlantic from sleeping sickness, this illness is caused by a kindred microorganism. This South and Central American version is typically carried by small house-infesting pests, sometimes called kissing bugs. The last thing you need is a "kiss" from one of these. They hide by day in wall cracks and linens. They feed by night. If a

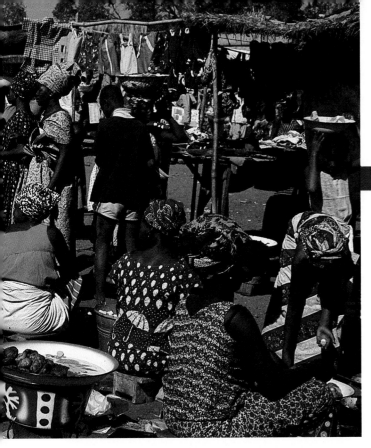

Vibrant colors, unusual foods and the hustle of merchants make this open market an exotic spot —but exotic spots such as these are also sometimes home to some fairly exotic diseases. In central Africa, where this picture was taken, tsetse flies carry the dreaded African sleeping sickness.

kissing bug carrying the loathsome *Trypanosoma cruzi* lands on your sleeping body, you may be in big trouble. How you do depends on which of the many strains of the organism got you (some are more dangerous than others), the condition of your immune system and the availability of proper medication. In the worst cases, your inner organs, particularly the esophagus and colon, can swell up much the way appendages do in elephantiasis victims.

Bolivian hemorrhagic fever. This is another disease that strikes in South America. Actually, it strikes only in rural areas of northeastern Bolivia, where the Machupo virus is rampant. Several epidemics over the past 25 years have devastated local villages. At least one village, El Mojon, suffered so severely that it has become a virtual ghost town. The virus is carried by a local mouselike rodent. It is believed that humans pick up the virus by coming into contact with the rodent's urine, either directly or through contaminated food and water. Victims of the virus suffer fever, abdominal pain and headaches. It can be fatal.

NORTHERN BLIGHTS

If you think all exotic diseases are found only in the tropics—think again. There are dozens of afflictions more common to temperate climates, sometimes found *only* in temperate climates, says Jack Poland, Ph.D., an epidemiologist and expert on rare infectious diseases.

Cystic hydatid disease. For centuries, this disease was a killer in one of the coldest of nations— Iceland. It is caused by a parasitic tapeworm often passed from sheep to dogs to their masters. It proved such a problem in sheep-filled Iceland that until only a few years ago, all dogs were banned from Reykjavik, the country's capital. The disease is still widespread in Yugoslavia, Bulgaria, Lebanon, Turkey and on the U.S. Navajo Indian reservation.

Colorado tick fever. Victims of this disease, which occurs only in the northwestern United States and western Canada, suffer severe headaches, soreness and high fever for up to ten days. "You feel like you're going to die, but you don't," says Dr. Poland. The disease, carried by the voracious *Dermacentor andersoni* tick, affects as many as 1,000 people a year.

Russian spring/summer encephalitis. This is another tick-borne disease, which may lead to more than a deathly feeling. Vomiting and headaches are only the beginning stages of this viral illness that often (about 40 percent of the time) leads to fatal inflammation of the brain and spinal cord. This affliction is most prevalent in mountainous areas of the Soviet Union and surrounding countries of Europe and Asia. There is nothing that can be done for victims but to try and keep them breathing until the infection passes on its own, says Dr. Poland.

Japanese encephalitis. This is a viral infection that is carried by mosquitoes throughout Southeast Asia. First discovered in Japan, then China, the deadly brain-attacking virus has since been well controlled in those countries through inoculation of children with a vaccine made mostly from mouse brain. In other Asian countries, such as India and Malaysia, where the vaccine is in short supply, the disease still ravages rural communities.

SELF-CARE FOR EVERYDAY INFECTIONS

Cavemen caught colds. Back then, if they wore down vests to keep out the chill, chances were the geese were still attached. Survival was *that* primitive.

Cavemen also carried brown clubs and brown sticks. But they didn't carry Blue Cross or Blue Shield. When they got sick they had to take care of themselves—a survival technique that has endured to this very day.

"Self-care is the original form of health care," says Lowell S. Levin, Ed.D., professor of public health, Yale University School of Medicine. "And it is still the primary source in health care. Nearly 90 percent of all health care today is people treating themselves."

SELF-CARE: THE BEST CARE

But are you in safe hands when you practice do-it-yourself health care? Dr. Levin believes you're in the *safest* hands—as long as you treat yourself intelligently.

"Self-care practices are tried and true," he says. "People won't continue a particular self-care approach to treat an ailment if they're finding it doesn't work. There's sort of a self-checking system that eliminates ineffective methods." But if it works, they'll try the method over and over again.

In fact, there is one particular self-care technique with a high success rate. It's called preventive self-care. And the strategy is simple: Take care of your immune system.

"If you have a prudent diet, try to minimize stress in your life, exercise and stop smoking, then your immune system will function at its optimum and help protect you from many everyday infections," says Gerald Hyner, Ph.D., professor of health education at Purdue University. It's the best self-care you can give yourself.

But no matter how well you take care of yourself,

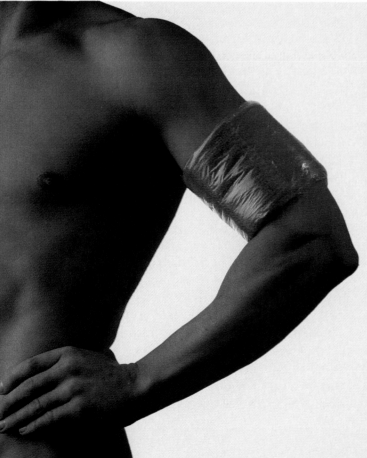

HOT PACKS HELP HEALING

Wounds heal more quickly when you turn up the heat, a University of California at San Francisco study indicates.

Researchers made hot packs out of wet towels sealed in plastic, then applied them to the upper arms of eight hospital patients. Using probes placed under the skin, they found that as temperature increased, so did the flow of oxygen to tissue. "Oxygen is very important in wound healing," says John Rabkin, M.D., a surgeon and coauthor of the study. The use of heat to aid healing is a "lost art," Dr. Rabkin says, although he cautions that it should be applied only after any swelling goes down. For years he's used hot packs to help infected incisions heal.

It works for little cuts and scrapes, too. "If you cut yourself, and the cut doesn't heal in a couple of days, put a hot pack, heating pad or warm towel on the area for a couple of hours while you watch TV," he suggests. "Do it two or three times and it's likely to help."

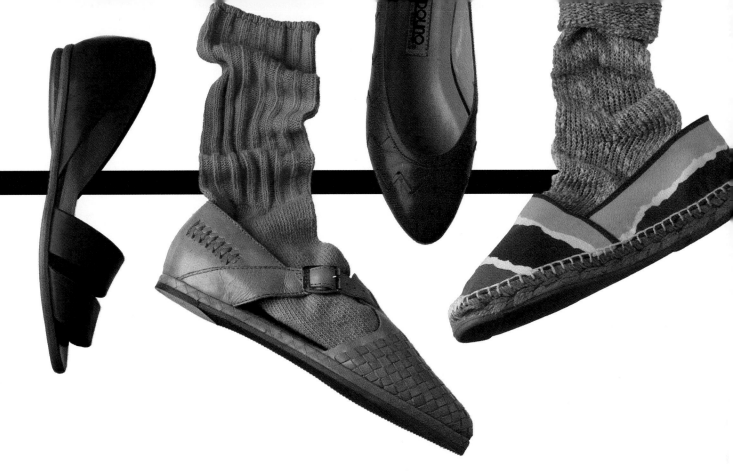

an infectious agent will sometimes take hold. When that happens, it's time to fight back with self-care. Here are the best self-care methods for the battle.

ATHLETE'S FOOT: HOW TO MAKE IT TOE THE LINE

You don't need to have athletic feet to get athlete's foot. As far as the fungus that causes it is concerned, any old kind of feet will do.

And when you get it, you *know* you've got it. Your feet may burn and peel. But most of all, they may itch. "You may feel it around the edges of the foot, on the sole of the foot, in between the toes," says Glenn Gastwirth, D.P.M., a podiatrist and director of scientific affairs for the American Podiatric Medical Association. And that itch will be so bad that you'll do almost anything to find relief. Fortunately, finding it is relatively simple.

Many over-the-counter athlete foot medications will work just fine if you follow the directions and use them properly, says Dr. Gastwirth. And he suggests another easy solution: letting your feet breathe a little.

"Create an inhospitable environment for the fungus by wearing shoes and socks that allow the feet to remain dry," he recommends. "Materials like leather and canvas allow moisture to escape and your feet to breathe."

Leather and canvas are the best shoe materials for preventing athlete's foot. Here are some other healthy foot tips from podiatrists. Buy shoes later in the day because as the day goes on, your feet swell and may be half a size larger than in the morning. For heels, the higher your age, the lower your heel should be, and because balance may be a problem when you get older, look for heels with a wider base.

You can also try drowning the fungus. Bathe your feet three to four times a week in warm water mixed with a half cup of vinegar, recommends Clare Starrett, D.P.M., of the Pennsylvania College of Podiatric Medicine. The acidity of the vinegar inhibits the fungus.

If you appear to have a stubborn case of athlete's foot—if it is still annoying you after ten days or so—Dr. Gastwirth suggests that you see your doctor. A prescription ointment may be your only solution.

A few simple preventive measures will help prevent you from having the problem again.

"Treat your feet like you do the rest of your body," says Dr. Gastwirth. "Bathe them, wash them with soap and dry them carefully after bathing. When you take a shower in a locker room or at a public pool, minimize your exposure to the fungus.

Wear rubber flip-flops or other foot coverings that you can wear in and out of the shower, and don't walk around barefoot."

CANKER SORES: THE INSIDE STORY

Canker sores are your mouth's way of biting you back. And they don't go about it subtly. One sip of lemonade or bite of a chili dog—Ouch! That stings! —can quickly confirm a diagnosis.

These sores can feel like giant craters but are actually miniature eruptions usually up to about $1/8$ inch in diameter. (Occasionally they *are* craters, getting as big as a inch in size!)

They are not contagious, but they do like movement. "Canker sores are much more likely to occur inside the mouth on the moveable tissue of the cheeks and tongue," says James Rooney, M.D., a senior staff fellow in the laboratory of oral medicine, National Institutes of Health (NIH).

Dr. Rooney says that the biochemical mechanics behind the formation of canker sores is unknown, but what starts the process is usually obvious—biting your cheek or tongue or injury to the tissue from hard-bristled toothbrushes or sharp-edged food like a corn chip. They're also known to occur during times of stress, after a fever or cold, or even after eating certain foods like chocolate, walnuts, citrus fruits, tomatoes or vinegar.

But canker sores could also be triggered by foods you're *not* eating. One study conducted by the NIH found that a diet deficient in iron, folate or vitamin B_{12} could bring on an attack. Thirty-nine patients who had recurrent episodes with canker sores were put on a diet high in these deficient nutrients. After six months, 23 of the patients were free of the sores.

Typically, says Dr. Rooney, a canker sore will run its course in about 10 to 14 days. He recommends using an over-the-counter topical anesthetic with benzocaine to help ease the pain. "Just dab it directly on the canker sore for relief," he says. "You can also buy gels that will cover the sore. It's good if you use them just before eating." You should also stay away from the hot and spicy foods that can fuel the pain.

If the pain becomes particularly severe, Dr. Rooney says it's a sign that the sore could be infected with bacteria. In such cases, your physician can prescribe tetracycline, an antibiotic that's been shown to reduce healing time, ulcer size and pain in canker sores.

COLD SORES:
HOW TO STOP THEM COLD

Cold sores aren't shy. Unlike canker sores, they don't hide in your mouth. Instead, they situate themselves around the mouth or lips where everybody can stare at them. Unlike canker sores, cold sores *are* contagious. *Very* contagious.

They're caused by a virus called herpes simplex. And if you've got it, you're not alone. "About 70 percent of the adult population over age 40 has been infected with herpes simplex virus," says Dr. Rooney. The majority of people infected, however, never have a problem with the disease.

Once the virus gets you, it never lets go. "People are infected for life," says Dr. Rooney. The virus hides away inside the nerve cells that sit just inside the base of your brain. It responds to certain conditions. Upper respiratory tract infections, fever, personal stress and overexposure to the sun are all common instigators. It also responds to an immune system that's on the blink. And, for some women, cold sores ride tandem with their menstrual cycles.

One way to put this virus on ice may be to use ice. One doctor, writing in the British medical journal *Lancet*, described dramatic results when his patients applied ice to their cold sores. Putting an ice pack directly on the sore continuously for 90 to 120 minutes can speed healing, reported Sanford Danziger, M.D., of the Department of Oral Medicine, Hebrew University/Hadassah Medical School in Jerusalem. If done within 24 hours of onset, he says, you should feel immediate relief from the pain and the blemish should disappear within one or two days.

FIRST PERSON REPORT:
COLD SORES

"I would like to pass along the best cure I know of for cold sores: Styptic pencil. I've been using this remedy for over 40 years. I moisten the pencil and apply it to the cold sore three or four times a day. The treatment clears up the problem and seems to prevent recurrence of infection."

I. H.
Racine, Wisconsin

Editor's Note: Styptic pencils are composed of two astringents, aluminum sulfate and aluminum chloride. These substances may help dry up cold sores but not necessarily stamp out the virus that causes them. In fact, styptic pencils can actually harbor the virus, causing further infection to the person using it. The American Dental Association cautions against using styptic pencils to treat cold sores.

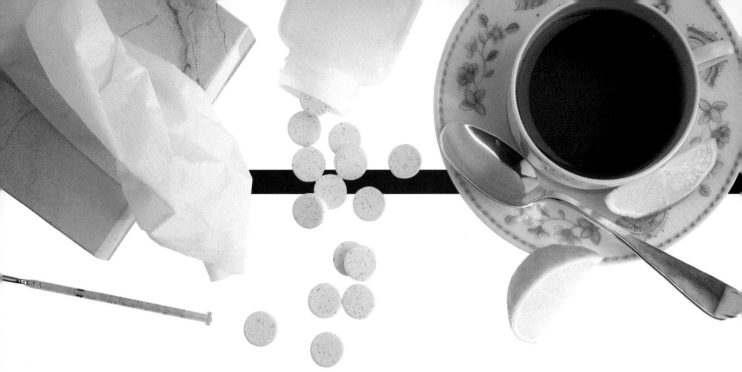

Generally, says Dr. Rooney, cold sores are most contagious "early on when they first form and are contagious as long as the blister has fluid in it, which is only the first couple of days."

Dr. Rooney recommends buying over-the-counter products like Blistex and Carmex that will dry out the sore. He also says to look for products with phenol, camphor or menthol, which have mild numbing and antiviral properties. If the OTC's don't work, Dr. Rooney recommends the prescription path. "Antiviral preparations work well with some people," he says. "Acyclovir, now available in cream form, can help the sore heal more quickly."

Dr. Rooney also reports that a recent study found that treating cold sores with the amino acid L-lysine showed favorable results when the patients took 1 gram three times a day. (Remember, however, that you should not take large amounts of this or any other nutritional supplement without the approval and supervision of your doctor.)

THE COMMON COLD: TIPS FOR COMFORT

There is nothing common about the common cold. In fact, there are so many bugs that cause it, they could have their own ZIP code. "What we call the cold is a condition that's caused by as many as 200 different viruses in four or five different virus families," says Jack Gwaltney, Jr., M.D., professor of medicine at the University of Virginia School of Medicine. The most common cold virus is the rhinovirus, which has scores of varieties of its own. It's no wonder a cold is so hard to kick!

From England to Texas, medical researchers report that using zinc to battle the common cold is nothing to sneeze at. England's Medical Research Council Common Cold Unit found that people who sucked zinc tablets reported less severe symptoms. At the University of Texas, researchers noted in a study, "Zinc lozenges shortened the average duration of colds by about seven days."

"No matter what you do to yourself, if a virus gets into your cells, and you're susceptible, you're going to catch a cold," says Helen Krause, M.D., chairman of the Immunology Committee of the American Academy of Otolaryngology-Head and Neck Surgery. "If you are exposed to a cold virus, like the rhinovirus, and you don't have the antibodies against that particular virus, then you're going to get sick."

There are two schools of thought as to how the notorious rhinovirus gets around. One belief is that it is spread through the air when a person coughs or sneezes. Elliot Dick, Ph.D., professor of preventive medicine at the University of Wisconsin Medical School, believes in this "aerosol" route and has done experiments that he says have stopped the virus in its tracks. They involved using a specially treated tissue, called a virucidal tissue, which can trap and kill the virus. "Blowing your nose carefully into a viricidal tissue and covering your mouth with it when you cough can be pretty effective against spreading a cold," he says.

Dr. Gwaltney suggests another possible route—the hand. "I don't know how colds are spread under natural conditions," he says. "But experiments suggest that colds can be spread by hand as well as through the air." And he says that it's probably the nose and eyes, not the mouth, that are the surest routes of entry. "Cold viruses don't grow well in the cells in your mouth."

In fact, kissing someone with a cold may be safer than rubbing noses. Dr. Dick conducted an experiment in which 16 healthy volunteers kissed people with colds, and only 1 of the volunteers came down with the virus.

No matter what the mode of transportation, most experts believe that good personal hygiene may be helpful in keeping cold viruses at bay. "Simply washing your hands often with soap and water removes the virus that's on your hands," says Dr. Gwaltney. "Unfortunately, it doesn't give you lasting protection."

All of which means, sooner or later, you're going to come down with a cold. What can you do to fight it?

Most physicians recommend that you treat your cold symptomatically. "Use an antihistamine if you have a runny nose and a decongestant like pseudo-ephedrine if you have a stuffy nose. Don't try to treat

symptoms that haven't appeared yet. The shotgun approach to treatment is not good treatment. This means you should stay away from multiple symptom products." (If you have heart disease, high blood pressure, asthma or glaucoma, or if you're pregnant or diabetic, you should consult your physician before using these products).

Over-the-counter nasal decongestants "work like adrenaline by tightening up the blood vessels," says David Fairbanks, M.D., an ear, nose and throat specialist in Washington, D.C. But he warns against using them for longer than three days. "You'll end up with rebound congestion," he says, meaning that

Rhinoviruses can't take the heat . . . at least that's the theory behind the Viralizer, a device that delivers a 120°F blast of medicated warm air to your nose. "Once the temperature inside your nose rises, the protein shell around the cold virus dissolves, and the virus dies," says Allan Aven, M.D., a family practitioner at Northwest Community Hospital in Arlington Heights, Illinois. Patients in a study who used the device to combat their colds showed surprising results."More than 90 percent got better in one or two days," Dr. Aven says.

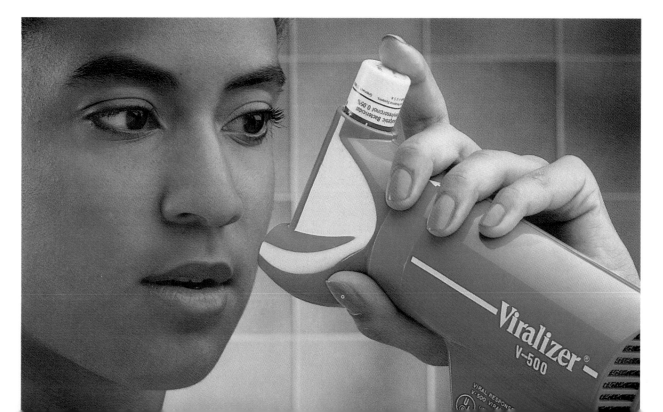

Editor's Note: These ingredients aren't on the roll call of the more scientifically tested cold remedies. But there are reasons to hope that someday garlic and vitamin C might be. Garlic has germicidal properties. And tomato juice and lemon juice contain vitamin C, which at least some evidence suggests may slightly reduce cold symptoms.

overuse of decongestants will actually *cause* congestion.

The stuffed-up feeling that's common with the common cold can be alleviated without medication, too. "The cold virus causes the blood vessels inside your nose to expand, and that leads to stuffiness," says Dr. Fairbanks. "When you lie down, the blood vessels act like varicose veins and fill up with blood." That's why sleeping is so difficult when you have a cold. He suggests that sleeping with your head higher than your heart will ease the discomfort. "Prop yourself up on a couple of pillows," he suggests.

A little dab of menthol can also bring some relief. "Menthol gives a sensation of coolness, and cold is a natural stimulus to open the nasal passage," says Dr. Fairbanks. "Put a little dab of some mentholated cold remedy under your nose."

He also says bundle up to keep your body—especially your feet—warm, but leave the temperature of the room air cool. This helps keep nasal passages open. Warm air contributes to stuffiness. "In the wintertime in heated homes, your nasal membranes become parched," he says. "A humidifier helps keep them moist and more able to resist infection better."

It's also important to keep the nasal mucus moving. Mucus stagnating in your nose, is a perfect place for a bacterial infection to take place," Dr. Fairbanks says. "When the mucus turns from clear to yellow or green and you start getting sinus pressure, it usually means your cold has developed into a secondary bacterial infection. When this happens you need to see a physician for an antibiotic prescription. It won't help get rid of the cold virus, but it will take care of the bacteria."

Another way to keep mucus flowing naturally is to drink plenty of hot liquids. In a study conducted at Mt. Sinai Medical Center in Miami Beach, researchers found that sipping hot water was more effective at loosening up nasal congestion than sipping cold water. But even more effective than hot water was hot chicken soup. According to the researchers, the vapor from the hot liquid is the secret to the soothing effect. How impressed were the Mt. Sinai researchers with the results? Well, the Mt. Sinai gift shop now markets its own brand of chicken soup!

CONJUNCTIVITIS: GETTING THE PINK OUT

"Conjunctivitis is inflammation of the white part of the eye," says Mitchell Friedlaender, M.D., director of the Cornea and External Diseases Division of Ophthalmology, Scripps Clinic and Research Foundation, La Jolla, California. "Your eye will turn red or pink, hence the term pinkeye. You'll notice either a watery or puslike discharge, and your eyelid will be sticky in the morning with crusting along the lashes. Your eye will also be sensitive to light, and you'll feel mild discomfort with a burning or itching feeling."

The most severe conjunctivitis is of the viral kind, caused by the adenovirus, but it can also be caused by an allergy, says Dr. Friedlaender. It's easy to distinguish between the two. "People usually know if they are allergic to pollen or cats," he says. "If when you come into contact with them and your eyes start to water or itch and become red, then that's pretty clearly an allergic conjunctivitis. Simply getting away from the allergen will make the conjunctivitis clear up."

Viral or bacterial conjunctivitis is a lot harder to deal with. For one thing, it can be very contagious. It's also very annoying.

Unfortunately, it usually requires a trip to the doctor to find out if your problem is being caused by a virus or bacteria. If a virus is the cause, you can expect the symptoms to last longer. There is no antidote; the problem simply has to run its course, which can take anywhere from one to two weeks.

Bacterial conjunctivitis, which can be diagnosed through a smear or culture, will clear up within five to seven days with a course of antibiotics.

Your best bet in dealing with conjunctivitis? Prevention.

"The virus is passed on through hand contact, so if you know of an outbreak or talk with someone who has a red, watery eye, make sure you wash your hands before touching your eye," says Dr. Friedlaender. "If someone comes down with it in your house, keep their towels and washcloths separate, along with anything else that they may come into contact with."

If you do come down with viral conjunctivitis, Dr. Friedlaender says that placing a hot or cold compress on the affected eye for a few minutes three or four times a day will help relieve some of the symptoms. Eyedrops sometimes will be prescribed. "They won't shorten the course of the disease or kill the virus," he says. "They just make the person feel better." You should also keep your hands away from your other eye to keep the disease from spreading.

CYSTITIS: DOUSING THE BURN

Twenty percent of all women in America will experience at least one bout of cystitis, which is an inflammation of the bladder. And they'll have no problem recognizing the symptoms. "Cystitis will burn when you pass urine and you'll feel like you have to urinate all the time," says Joseph Corriere, M.D., professor and director of urology at the University of Texas Medical School. "A burning feeling in the urinary area will wake you up at night, and many times you will even have blood in your urine."

The most common cause of cystitis in young females is the introduction of bacteria through the urethra and into the bladder during sexual intercourse, says Dr. Corriere. Another cause is vaginal infection. Some 5 percent of women with cystitis will have a vaginal infection. And, he says, women who have infections during their menstrual periods may decrease their risk of developing cystitis by using pads rather than tampons.

Although the evidence is inconclusive, some experts believe that eating certain foods may aggravate cystitis. Foods like citrus fruit, spices, coffee and alcohol may raise the acid level and stimulate the production of bacterial growth. The result? A burning in the bladder.

One way it's thought that women can help prevent the infection is to always wipe themselves from front to back. Another is to avoid tight jeans and panty hose and undergarments without a cotton crotch, all of which create a perfect environment for the bacteria to thrive. Women who are prone to the disease should also drink plenty of liquids and empty their bladder after intercourse to help flush microorganisms out of their systems.

The most effective way to stop an inflammation already in progress, however, is a course of antibiotics. Dr. Corriere recommends the antibiotic nitrofurantoin macrocrystals, which doesn't upset the delicate balance of helpful bacteria in the bowel and vagina as do some other antibiotics.

And what about cranberry juice, a folk remedy often touted as a preventive and cure? Well, you can give it a try, but don't be disappointed if it doesn't do you a whole lot of good.

"It's true that cranberry juice has the ability to acidify urine, but someone with the infection can't keep it in the bladder long enough for it to acidify," says Richard Szabo, M.D., a urologist at Kaiser-Permanente in San Francisco. "Cranberry juice makes sense in a test tube, but in the body it gets flushed out too fast."

FEVER: RISING TO THE OCCASION

Your immune system is in favor of the death penalty. Any virus or bacterium convicted of causing disease is likely to be fried.

"An infection stimulates the immune system," says Donna McCarthy, Ph.D., assistant professor of nursing, University of Wisconsin, Madison, School of Nursing, and an expert on the role fever plays in dealing with infection. "The immune system then signals the brain that it would like a warmer body temperature because the immune cells that attack the actual infecting organism work more efficiently at a higher temperature. So it's a nice circuit: The infection activates the immune cells, those cells signal the brain, the brain raises the body temperature and that makes it easier for the immune cells to operate."

So a fever is actually a *good* sign—a sign that your immune system is working to get rid of a body invader. But that's the only good thing about it. When you get a fever, you generally feel really bad. But Dr. McCarthy believes there's good reason for this.

"The same system that signals your brain to raise your body temperature also acts to stimulate sleep," says Dr. McCarthy. "So it's good for you to rest when you have a temperature. Your body wants to conserve energy to fight the infection."

Fever can cause a secondary problem, though: dehydration. But it can be avoided by replacing the fluids that are lost through "invisible" perspiration, says David Sobel, M.D., regional director of patient education at Kaiser-Permanente in San Jose, California.

Self-care advice applies mainly to fevers below 103°F in someone under the age of 60 who is otherwise in good health. But the older you get, the more attention you should pay to a fever. Research has found that the closer your age gets to your temperature reading, the more serious having a fever becomes.

This is what doctors at Hartford Hospital, an emergency room/walk-in clinic in Connecticut, discovered in a study of 1,200 people who came to the hospital with a fever of 101°F or more. Of those between the ages of 17 to 39, the doctors found that in more than 50 percent of the cases, the fever was associated with a common viral problem, such as a sore throat. In patients over age 60, however, only 4 percent were suffering from mild illnesses. In fact, in more than 90 percent of the cases, the patients had to be hospitalized. They were found to have more serious illnesses, such as bacterial pneumonia or inflammation of the gallbladder or digestive tract.

"If you're over the age of 60 and your temperature is over 102°F, you should call your doctor immediately," says Herbert Keating, M.D., the leading researcher on the study, who is chairman of the Department of Medicine at the Medical Center of Delaware. "Any fever in a person 60 or 65 years of age can be a serious problem."

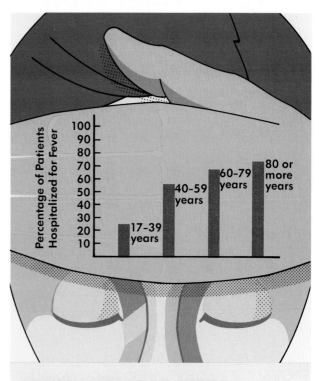

FEVER: DANGER RISES WITH AGE

Hospital emergency rooms admit older people with temperatures at a more feverish pace than they do younger people. At least that's what a study at one New England hospital found. More than 70 percent of those over age 80 were admitted—usually with suspected serious illness—as compared with less than 30 percent of the people aged 17 to 39. The younger patients, for the most part, had common viral problems such as colds and sore throats.

Experts also recommend that, no matter what your age, you should call your physician if you have a temperature over 103°F, if the fever you have lasts more than three days, if it's accompanied by rash, severe headache, stiff neck, confusion, back pain or painful urination, or if you have diabetes, heart or lung disease.

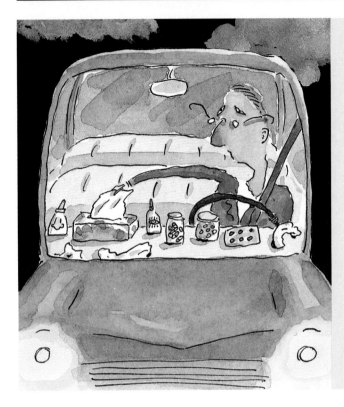

DRIVING UNDER THE INFLUENZA

Don't be caught DWI. Those letters could just as easily stand for "driving with influenza" as for their usual meaning, "driving while intoxicated."

Researchers in England measured the hand/eye coordination and reaction speed of volunteers who were ailing with either a cold or the flu.

The cold sufferers flew through the reaction test, but the flu sufferers hit the brakes, *slowly*. Their reaction times were down 57 percent, compared with the 5 to 10 percent reduction that occurs when a person consumes a couple of alcoholic drinks.

It seems that you should be more careful coming down the road if you're coming down with the flu.

THE FLU: HOW TO STOP IT FROM BUGGING YOU

"Influenza is a viral infection that may also affect the lower respiratory tract," says Thomas Torok, M.D., a medical epidemiologist who specializes in influenza at the Centers for Disease Control (CDC) in Atlanta. "Classically, infection consists of fever, cough, headache and muscle ache. Signs of upper respiratory tract illness like a stuffy or runny nose are also common. It does not make you sick to your stomach, though, as many people think."

Like Christmas, the flu is an annual event, striking worldwide, usually around the last part of January or first part of February. Luckily, you can revoke the passport of this jet-setter. There is both a prescription medication and a vaccination to prevent the flu.

The pill, called amantadine hydrochloride, has been found effective against the disease, but it definitely has its drawbacks, says Dr. Torok. "The medi-

cine has to be taken once or twice a day for as long as the influenza is present in your community, which could be as long as several months," he says. "It's expensive, and it only works against certain strains. Also, it has side effects, especially in elderly people." The flu vaccination is a more common choice. "The vaccine is the best way to protect yourself against the flu," says Dr. Torok.

The reason there's a vaccine against the flu virus and not the cold virus is because the flu doesn't have hundreds of forms like the cold bug does. But it is sneakier.

"Currently there are three strains of influenza circulating, and they change slightly in genetic makeup from year to year," says Dr. Torok. "So we annually update the flu vaccination to have it more closely match the virus that's here this year." That's also why the flu shot that took care of you last year won't protect you this year.

Who should get flu shots? "If you have chronic

heart and lung disease, you may be more susceptible to catching the flu and developing serious complications from it. Elderly people in nursing homes, or even healthy people over 65, should make sure they get the vaccination every year," says Dr. Torok.

An inoculation can help even if you've already caught the flu. "You need to protect yourself from other strains that may be circulating," says Dr. Torok. "You may have influenza a, but the vaccine could protect you from coming down with influenza b. Also, if you take amantadine within 48 hours of onset, it can modify the course of the illness and reduce the severity of symptoms."

The infection should last five to seven days, but it is not unusual to feel washed out from the bout for up to two weeks, notes Dr. Torok. Physicians recommend resting in bed for the first few days, drinking plenty of fluids and taking aspirin or acetaminophen to relieve the aches and pains. (Children with fevers should never take aspirin, because of the risk of Reye's syndrome. For more information, see the box "Every Parent's Nightmare" on page 13.)

A FLU SHOT "BOOSTER"

It's time to needle you about eating right, because good nutrition can give you a better shot at avoiding the flu, even if you've had a protective flu shot.

After Canadian researchers gave a flu vaccine to 30 malnourished elderly patients, they divided them into two groups. One group was taught to eat more nutritiously and also received supplements. After four weeks, those patients had significantly more antibodies to the flu virus than the group whose nutrition wasn't improved.

"The correction of . . . undernutrition in the elderly may be expected to improve immune responses," the researchers concluded, "and perhaps result in better protective immunity."

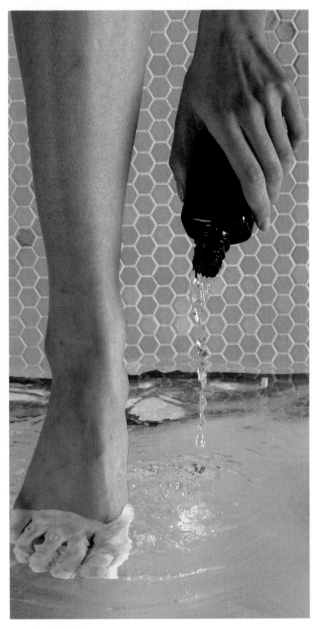

A nice, warm vinegar footbath is a great way to beat bacteria-caused foot odor and to soothe your aching feet. But if you see an ingrown toenail brewing, make some black tea and steep your feet in it twice a day for 5 to 10 minutes. The tannic acid in tea has a drying effect, and dry skin resists ingrown nail penetration better than moist skin.

FOOT ODOR: THE SECRET OF SWEET FEET

It's normal for your feet to have an odor. But if slipping off your shoes makes others want to leave the room, you might have a foot odor problem.

Foot odors are caused by bacteria decomposing in perspiration. So if your feet sweat a lot, they probably will smell a lot. Reducing the perspiration, then, is the key to clearing the air around your feet.

"Wear socks made of natural materials that absorb moisture or move it away from your feet," recommends Dr. Gastwirth. Foot powder containing aluminum chlorhydrate also may help keep your skin dry, but you should sprinkle it on lightly. "Too much powder tends to become a paste, which can block the pores and may actually make the problem worse," says Dr. Gastwirth.

If the odor is still a problem, Dr. Gastwirth advises changing your shoes and socks at least twice a day. And make sure what you change into is clean and dry.

GINGIVITIS: TIPS FOR HEALTHIER GUMS

If sore, bleeding gums and bad breath are plaguing you, it's likely you've got gingivitis, an ominous sign of bigger and badder things to come.

"Gingivitis is an inflammation of your gums," says Steven Budnick, D.D.S., associate professor of oral pathology at Emory University. "Your gums turn from pink to bright red and become puffy and bleed when you brush or floss. It's caused by plaque and microorganisms that get on your teeth and harden under your gums into a substance called dental calculus." If not taken care of, gingivitis can gradually lead to periodontal disease, a painful condition that can result in tooth loss.

But you can reverse gingivitis. All it takes is good oral hygiene—which is the same thing that prevents it from happening in the first place.

What's required? "Daily brushing (at least twice a day), flossing, and seeing your dentist twice a year will take care of it for most people," says Dr. Budnick.

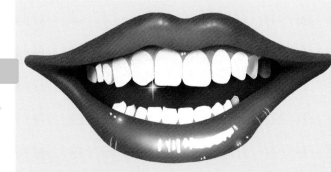

VITAMIN C
TAKES THE BITE
OUT OF GINGIVITIS

Adequate vitamin C intake may play a key role in the early stages of gum disease. In a study done at the University of California, San Francisco, School of Dentistry and reported in the *Journal of Periodontology,* researchers found that gingivitis increased when volunteers were deprived of vitamin C, then decreased significantly when their diets were supplemented with the nutrient.

The volunteers were fed a diet that gave them all the nutrients they required except for vitamin C. For the first two weeks of the study, they received oral doses of 60 milligrams a day (the Recommended Dietary Allowance) of the vitamin, which brought them all to the same baseline level.

During the following four weeks, the volunteers received a look-alike placebo instead of the vitamin. For three weeks after that, they got a 600-milligram dose of C, followed once again by a four-week placebo period.

Although the volunteers showed no signs of serious gum disease during the period when they were vitamin C deficient, they did have far more inflammation and bleeding during that time than during the period when they took the supplements.

Also, they reported that the bleeding and inflammation subsided significantly when they returned to taking vitamin C daily.

"Toothpaste and mouthwashes with plaque-fighting agents help, but they only work with plaque above the gums, so it's important that people still floss. If you're showing signs of gingivitis, these measures will, in time, remove all the irritants under the gum, and the bleeding will stop."

Sometimes, however, the inflammation known as gingivitis will turn into the infection known as trench mouth. At this point, consider your problem very serious.

Trench mouth, clinically known as acute necrotizing ulcerative gingivitis, causes rotting of the gums, especially the points of the gums between the teeth. Its symptoms are painful swollen gums, a metallic taste in the mouth and severe bad breath.

And it's not just bad health habits that can cause it. Stress can also be to blame. "It affects people whose immune systems aren't functioning properly because they're run-down from not eating or sleeping right," says Dr. Budnick. "This, combined with improper oral care, gives the bacteria a perfect environment in which to grow."

Because it's a bacterial infection, antibiotics work well to fight it. A healthy eating plan is also recommended, along with a good, thorough clean-

ing and plenty of attention by a dentist. "Changing your lifestyle and slowing down a bit wouldn't hurt either," notes Dr. Budnick.

HERPES SIMPLEX II:
DEALING WITH A DELICATE PROBLEM

"From 1966 to 1984 the number of physician/patient consultations for genital herpes increased 15 times," says Thomas Becker, M.D., an epidemiologist and assistant professor of medicine at the University of New Mexico School of Medicine. In one recent year, it was estimated that 470,000 people in the United States were treated for the virus for the first time. And the numbers continue to grow.

"If you've got it, you're certainly not alone," says Stephen Straus, M.D., head of medical virology at the National Institute of Allergy and Infectious Diseases. "Twenty to 40 percent of the adults in the United States carry the virus. But only a minority of people who have the virus have frequent outbreaks. Most are so mildly affected, they aren't even aware they have the disease."

Symptoms of the virus range from fever and chills with a flulike syndrome to small, fluid-filled lesions that appear on the penis or in and around the vagina. When these lesions rupture, they become infected, and this can cause itching, burning and general discomfort in the genital area.

Dr. Straus says that his own research has shown that herpes can be passed to another person from someone who has the disease but isn't experiencing overt symptoms. "It's probably one of the major ways in which it is spread," says Dr. Straus. "Even if no lesions or other symptoms are present, a partner of a herpes sufferer is still at risk for getting it."

George Schmid, M.D., a clinical researcher in the Division of Sexually Transmitted Diseases at the CDC, agrees. "Most people who've acquired the herpes simplex II infection presume that they got it from a socially unconscionable individual who had overt symptoms and didn't say anything. But that is not really the case."

Dr. Schmid says that there have been two studies done that confirm this perspective. "In one study, the researchers discovered that two-thirds of the individuals who passed on infections had no symptoms or did not recognize their symptoms at the time of transmission," he says.

Other researchers discovered something else.

"They found the herpes simplex virus on the penile or vaginal skin of those who had no visible lesions," he says.

As a result, many doctors recommend that those with the virus use barrier methods at all times during sex. "We recommend you use a lubricated condom so you have a mechanical barrier [the condom], and a chemical barrier [the spermicide]," says Denise Buntin, M.D., associate professor of dermatology at the University of Tennessee Health Science Center in Memphis. "Studies have shown that spermicides can kill the herpes virus."

She also recommends that latex condoms be used. "Studies have shown that the herpes virus can go through a condom made of animal skin, but it can't go through a latex one," she says.

Fortunately for herpes sufferers, there is now drug therapy available that will help relieve the painful symptoms, although it will not get rid of the disease permanently.

"Acyclovir [sold as Zovirax] is unquestionably an effective drug," says Dr. Straus, who has researched its use in treating genital herpes. "It's not a cure, but it lessens the severity of first-time episodes. It also

"Lysine appears to be an effective agent for reduction of occurrence, severity and healing time for recurrent herpes simplex infections," say researchers at the Indiana University School of Medicine. Study participants took 1,000 milligrams of the amino acid lysine three times a day for six months. More than 60 percent experienced improvement.

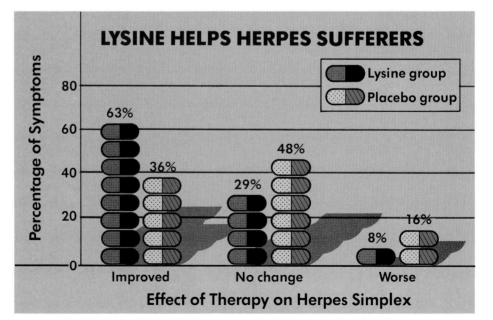

134

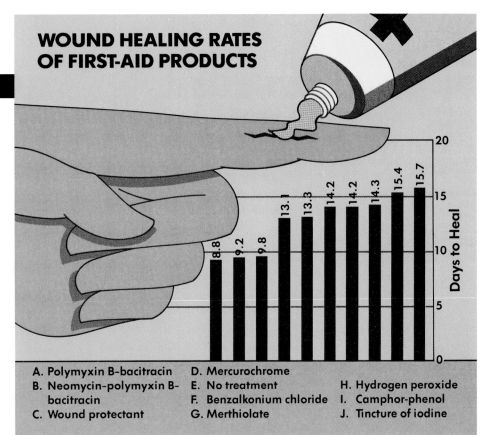

WOUND HEALING RATES OF FIRST-AID PRODUCTS

Treating wounds with antibiotic ointments helps speed up the healing process, a study by James Leyden, M.D., showed. Polymyxin B-bacitracin (available over the counter as Polysporin) and neomycin-polymyxin B-bacitracin (available as Neosporin) were the fastest healer/helpers of all.

Days to Heal: 8.8, 9.2, 9.8, 13.1, 13.3, 14.2, 14.2, 14.3, 15.4, 15.7

A. Polymyxin B-bacitracin
B. Neomycin-polymyxin B-bacitracin
C. Wound protectant
D. Mercurochrome
E. No treatment
F. Benzalkonium chloride
G. Merthiolate
H. Hydrogen peroxide
I. Camphor-phenol
J. Tincture of iodine

helps a little bit with recurrences. People can stay on it for months at a time, and it dramatically reduces recurrences. It doesn't have many side effects. For people who have frequent trouble with infections, acyclovir makes a big difference."

In addition to drug therapy, there are also a few self-help measures that can help relieve the pain of herpes lesions, says Janet Kreitman, coordinator of the Herpes Resource Center of the American Social Health Assocation.

"A sitz bath, which consists of soaking the pelvic area in warm, hip-high water, can help a person with herpes feel more comfortable," she says. "If the lesions are very painful, use a hair dryer on a low setting to dry the affected skin."

Kreitman says it's highly unlikely that the virus can be spread on towels, "but it's a good idea not to share towels in the small likelihood that there is live virus on them."

She stresses, though, that people should not use petroleum jelly on herpes sores. "It's possible to spread the lesions even more by doing that," she says. "It's also not a good idea to pop the blisters,

because that increases the chances of spreading."

Aspirin may also help relieve the pain. And, says Kreitman, women who have herpes should have a Pap smear at least twice a year. "It's still unknown if there is a link between cervical cancer and herpes," she says.

And what's her advice to avoid recurrences? "At the center's hotline [(415) 328-7710], we tell people to take care of their health—try to avoid stress, live a balanced life and have a good diet," she says.

INFECTED CUTS AND BURNS: TREATMENT AND PREVENTION

Ouch! A minor cut or burn causes a moment of pain. But if the sore is still hurting after a day or two, consider it the first sign of infection.

"Pain is the earliest symptom of a cut that's become infected," says Keith Sivertson, M.D., director of the Department of Emergency Medicine at Johns Hopkins Hospital in Baltimore. "Twenty-four to 30 hours after an injury is when you reach maximum soreness. If on the second or third day the wound is still getting more painful, you have to be

SQUELCHING SHINGLES PAIN

Shingles is chicken pox grown up. If you thought the chicken pox virus flew the coop long ago when you were young, you're wrong. Ninety percent of the people who ever had chicken pox still have the herpes zoster virus in their bodies.

It's a virus that lies dormant in the nerve cells that line the spinal column and brain. Suddenly, decades later, it may awake and attack. "When people live long enough, they seem to outgrow the immunity they had to this disease," says Leon Robb, M.D., an anesthesiologist who specializes in pain management at Hollywood Presbyterian Medical Center. "The person then gets severe pain following along the affected nerve and a localized florid rash that looks just like chicken pox."

Although the disease mostly strikes older people, Dr. Robb says, "Now we're seeing it in younger people who are immune-compromised—people with AIDS or cancer patients who are on drugs that suppress their immune systems."

"If we see the patient in the first month, we can inject medicine that blocks the sympathetic nerve, which in turn shuts off the pain cycle. That brings dramatic results. Well over 90 percent of the patients feel relief." Along with the nerve block, Dr. Robb advises his patients to take 375 milligrams of L-lysine (an amino acid) four times a day.

Other researchers are finding out that spice can make you feel nice. David Bickers, M.D., professor of dermatology at Case Western Reserve University School of Medicine, reports that a cream made with capsaicin (a compound derived from hot red peppers) provided "substantial relief" from lingering shingles pain. Dr. Bickers had patients apply the cream five times a day for one week, then three times a day after that. After four weeks of treatment, 75 percent of the patients reported being pain free. Zostrix, a topical analgesic cream containing capsaicin, is available at pharmacies.

---

worried that the wound is infected."

Your worries will soon be confirmed, not by what you feel but by what you see. "Redness is the second sign," he says. "Inflammation, seen as redness and swelling, means white blood cells are swarming to the site of the infection."

If you see redness and feel increased pain, an over-the-counter antibacterial cream such as Bacitracin may help stop an infection early on. If the pain, redness and swelling become more intense and the wound begins to drain, however, consider the infection in progress. And consider progressing to your doctor.

"Chances are the infection may be the result of a foreign body such as dirt, a splinter or glass in the wound that needs to be removed," says Dr. Sivertson. "Also, you need to find out if the infection is spreading beyond the wound." The treatment of choice?

Antibiotics such as penicillin or tetracycline will usually clear up an infection in a matter of days.

Burns also hurt when they get infected. But unlike cuts, you won't see any pus, says Terry Housinger, M.D., assistant chief of staff at the Shriner's Burn Institute of the University of Cincinnati. "The skin and tissue right under the burn become infected often by the same organisms that cause an abscess and draining in a cut."

But as with cuts, redness and increased pain *are* signs of an infected burn. "There will be redness surrounding the burn, maybe a little more redness in the burn itself, and the area will be tender," says Dr. Housinger. Again, an over-the-counter antibacterial cream may help stave off an early infection. If the symptoms don't decrease within 24 hours, see your doctor. Most burns that you can care for yourself should heal within one to two weeks, he notes.

An infection is merely the result of the immune system losing a battle with a bacterial enemy that entered your body through the open wound. Stop it at the point of entry and you can keep an infection from ever happening.

"In the case of a cut, let the wound bleed, then wash it immediately with soap and water," advises Dr. Sivertson. "Keep it clean and dry. And, if you can, keep it open to the air."

Your age and the location of the wound are also important healing factors. "The younger you are, the more quickly a wound will heal," he says. Generally, wounds that don't get infected will heal completely in about 20 to 25 days (longer if the cut is over a joint such as the knuckle or knee). But research is showing that you may be able to speed up the process. Antibiotic first-aid creams help heal wounds faster, according to James Leyden, M.D., professor of dermatology at the University of Pennsylvania.

If you're choosing a first-aid ointment, Dr. Leyden recommends looking for one containing antibiotics. "They will kill the bacteria but not have an adverse effect on the healing process. Antimicrobial antiseptics like iodine or hydrogen peroxide kill the bacteria but seem to also have a negative effect on healing. They're not as gentle to the wound and aren't as good at wound healing as an antibiotic."

To prevent a burn from getting infected, Dr. Leyden suggests washing it immediately with warm water, then applying an over-the-counter antibiotic ointment. "Wash it a couple of times a day with a gentle soap to keep it clean," he says, "and if you can, leave it open to the air. If, however, there's a chance it can get dirty, cover it with gauze."

SINUS INFECTIONS: RELIEF FOR FLARE-UPS

An unfortunate 30 to 50 million people experience the wrath of periodic sinus flare-ups, making sinusitis one of the five most common "minor" health complaints in the country. When you have it, though, the symptoms feel anything but minor.

"Bacterial sinusitis shows up as head pain, facial tenderness over the affected sinus, yellow or green drainage from the nose or down the back of the throat, and sometimes fever," explains Steven Schaefer, M.D., professor of head and neck surgery in the Department of Otolaryngology at the University of Texas Health Science Center at Dallas.

Viruses can also provoke a sinus outburst. "Remember the last time you caught a cold? Chances

IS IT REALLY YOUR SINUSES?

Many people dub themselves sinus sufferers, when actually they've got something else that mimics a sinus problem. Knowing the difference is crucial, because treatments aren't always the same.

The allergic condition known as hay fever is an example. The nasal lining of a person with hay fever becomes inflamed, causing sinusitislike symptoms such as a runny or clogged nose. Since some of the same nerves serve the nose and sinuses, it's easy to see why someone might come up with an inaccurate self-diagnosis of sinus problems. In this case, treating the allergy is essential.

True sinus trouble involves one or more of four sets of cranial cavities that compose the paranasal sinuses. You have one set, called *frontal* sinuses, in the brow area over your eyes. Inside each cheekbone are your *maxillary* sinuses. Your *sphenoid* sinuses are in the upper region, deep inside, behind your nose. And your *ethmoidal* sinuses, troublemakers that are more like small bunches of grapes rather than two distinct cavities, are behind the bridge of your nose.

The sinuses, passageways and nasal walls are lined with mucous membranes. A normal day's work for these structures finds air and secretions flowing easily from the sinuses, through the tunnels and out the nose. When something interferes with this process, sinus trouble begins.

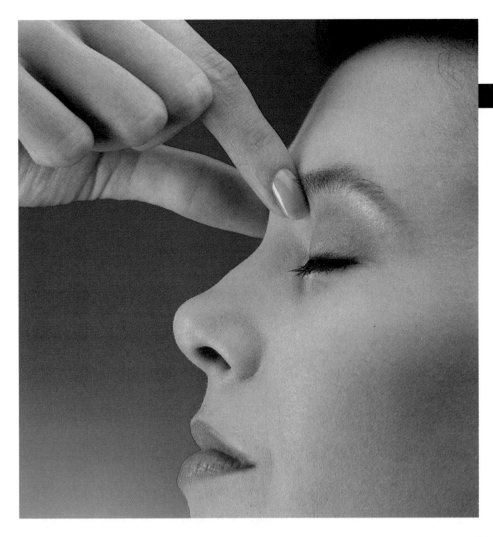

For sinus relief, try acupressure, the oriental medical art. Here's the technique: With your thumbs or fingertips, press and massage the areas right under your eyebrows that are in line with the sinus area. Move in firm, slow circles, stop, and repeat.

are the virus that nabbed you first appeared as a stuffy nose with clear, runny mucus, and then things turned ugly—yellow or green secretions, postnasal drip, a slight fever," says Bruce Jafek, M.D., chairman of the Department of Otolaryngology/Head and Neck Surgery at the University of Colorado School of Medicine. "This is secondary bacterial overgrowth. It's quite a pain in the head while you have it, but it tends to get better in time on its own."

Acute attacks of sinusitis may last from a day to a month. Chronic conditions, while usually not as painful, may hang on indefinitely.

If you're susceptible, there's really no way to prevent all future assaults of sinusitis. But you *don't* have to be stuck under a sinus siege that drags on and on. Here's what you need to know for next time:
● Learn the dos and don'ts of blowing your nose. "If you sound like a mating elk, you're blowing too hard," says Dr. Jafek. "Too much force creates pres-

sure in your nose that will push bacteria and pathogens up into your sinuses. Blow gently with both nostrils, never one at a time."
● Use decongestants for relief. Over-the-counter sinus relief products can help unclog you, and unclogging will ease the pain. (Over-the-counter pain relievers can also soften your headache, but they won't help get rid of what's bugging you.) Follow the directions on the package carefully.
● Don't rely on nasal sprays. They do provide temporary relief, but repeated use can eventually paralyze the tiny "sweeper" hairs, or cilia, that normally give the brush-off to infection-causing dirt and bacteria.
● For the same cilia-damaging reasons, stop smoking once and for all. And avoid rooms crawling with puffers.
● Resist the urge to retreat to bed. It's probably the first place you'll want to go during a bad attack, but sinus pain is even more powerful when you're prone.

Likewise, ever notice that when you bend over, your head feels like a towel being rung out? The most comfortable position, and one that encourages nasal drainage, is sitting upright and leaning slightly forward, as if you're writing a letter at your desk.

• Invest in a humidifier for your home if the air is dry. Moist nasal membranes help keep viruses and bacteria away from your sinus cavities. Electrostatic air filters screen irritating particles and are worthwhile, too.

If these measures don't help, and you have a fever or severe pain, you need to be seen by a physician, who will probably prescribe antibiotics if you have an infection, and will search for the cause of your condition.

If you suspect that allergies are instigating your sinus problems, your doctor can test for specific things to which your system reacts. Antihistamines and other medications, or a series of immunity-building shots, might bring your allergies—and as a result, your sinus problems—to heel.

SORE THROAT: PUTTING THE FIRE OUT

Does your throat feel like you've spent the last 15 years as a sword swallower in a side show? Does it hurt so much that you even cringe at the thought of swallowing your pride?

If you don't own a sword, it's a pretty safe bet that your sore throat is being caused by a viral or bacterial infection. (Allergies can bring on a sore throat, but there will be other symptoms, such as a runny nose and itchy, watery eyes.)

To confirm your suspicions, step up to the bathroom mirror and say "ahhhhhh." "Look to see if your throat is red and if there is pus on your tonsils," says John Middelkamp, M.D., professor of pediatrics at Washington University School of Medicine. "Also check to see if there are little red or white dots on your soft palate or roof of your mouth. Check to see if the glands on the side of your neck are tender and swollen. If you have all these symptoms, and a fever, you probably have a strep infection."

A sore throat is never a thing you should take lightly, says Dr. Middlekamp. If it's strep and goes undetected, he notes, it could lead to rheumatic fever, which is a serious infection of the joints and heart muscle and valves.

Most of the time, however, your sore throat will not be strep, and your own self-treatment can help soothe the pain and make you feel better within 48 hours. Dr. Sobel recommends the following measures:

• Drink at least six glasses of fluids daily. It will help keep the throat moist and reduce the pain.

• Gargle several times daily with warm saltwater. About ¼ teaspoon of salt in 4 ounces of water is good.

• Suck on hard candy, cough drops or lozenges to moisten and soothe the throat.

• Take aspirin or acetaminophen as needed to alleviate the pain.

• If you're a smoker, stop. Smoking irritates the throat.

INSTANT SORE THROAT RELIEF

Lozenges, gargles or sprays do not kill cold viruses or speed healing, but they may provide temporary relief from minor throat pain.

The following anesthetics have been proved safe and effective for cold-related sore throats:

• Benzocaine—found in Children's Chloraseptic and Spec-T Sore Throat Anesthetic lozenges.

• Hexylresorcinol—found in Sucrets lozenges.

• Phenol (Sodium phenolate) found in Chloraseptic lozenges.

• Dyclonine hydrochloride.

• Salicyl alcohol.

• Benzyl alcohol.

In lozenges, these drugs typically begin to work within 1 to 5 minutes and provide relief for up to 30 minutes. The Food and Drug Administration recommends against using them continuously for more than two days.

WARTS: TWO SIMPLE SOLUTIONS

Kissing a frog may get you a prince, but it won't give you warts. "Warts are caused by the human papilloma virus," says Thomas Flanagan, Ph.D., a virologist and professor of microbiology at the State University of New York at Buffalo School of Medicine. "There are at least 16 different types of these viruses, and some of the types are associated with warts in different anatomical locations." In other words, some wart viruses have a thing for feet; others like hands. And some might just have a preference for the tip of your nose.

If you have caught the virus, you can do something or you can do nothing. First, the nothing. "A great number of warts—probably 70 percent of them—will go away on their own within a two-year period," says John Romano, M.D., a dermatologist and professor at New York Hospital/Cornell Medical Center.

If the wart happens to be caused by the kind of virus that prefers the tip of your little finger, and you don't feel like leaving it there for two years, Dr. Romano recommends using an over-the-counter preparation with salicylic acid in it. "The acid doesn't kill the virus, but it causes an inflammation to occur. When that happens, white blood cells come to the site of the inflammation and then they produce the proper substances to get rid of the wart."

Now for the something: vitamin A. In studies done at Tulane University School of Medicine, virologist Robert F. Garry, Ph.D., discovered that "applying vitamin A got rid of common warts in about a month and a half to five months.

"You don't need to swallow the vitamin A capsule," he says. "Open the capsule up and rub the contents on the wart. Rub it on once a day, then wipe the excess off and leave the wart open to the air."

YEAST INFECTIONS: STOPPING RECURRENCES

A yeast infection or vaginitis is a common curse that causes itching, burning and a malodorous discharge from the vagina. Its most common cause is a one-celled fungus called *Candida*. And although only women are plagued with its chronic symptoms, men can carry the fungus, too.

In fact, in some cases, men are actually the cause of the problem. They pass it onto their partner during sex. "Almost always, when you have chronic *Candida* infections, you'll find that the male has yeast in his mouth or ejaculate," says Benson Horowitz, M.D., a vulvologist and associate clinical professor of obstetrics and gynecology at the University of Connecticut School of Medicine. "A man doesn't know he has it because he doesn't suffer any of the symptoms, but when he gives it to a woman it results in an infection, creating the itching and burning. This is why often the male as well as a female in a relationship should be cultured and treated."

But sex is not the only vehicle responsible for yeast infections. Women are quite capable of infecting themselves. "Yeast is a common inhabitant of the gastrointestinal tract, so most people have yeast in their rectums," says Howard Kent, M.D., director of medical education and associate professor of obstetrics and gynecology at Jefferson Medical College, Thomas Jefferson University. "In the summertime, when most yeast infections occur, you see women walking around in wet bathing suits. The yeast can migrate from the rectum to the vagina through the wet material."

No matter how you've developed this pesky problem, there are some things you can do for yourself to help get rid of the problem and discourage a recurrence.

Taking a sitz bath, preferably a bath in a solution of salt and water, will help cut down the invading bacteria and help ease the maddening itch, say doctors. You should also practice good hygiene. Always keep the vaginal area clean and dry and avoid wearing tight jeans and panty hose. You want to keep the area cool and airy.

Simple carbohydrates—sugary foods, wine and alcohol—are believed to create a sugar overload that contributes to an unhealthy vaginal environment.

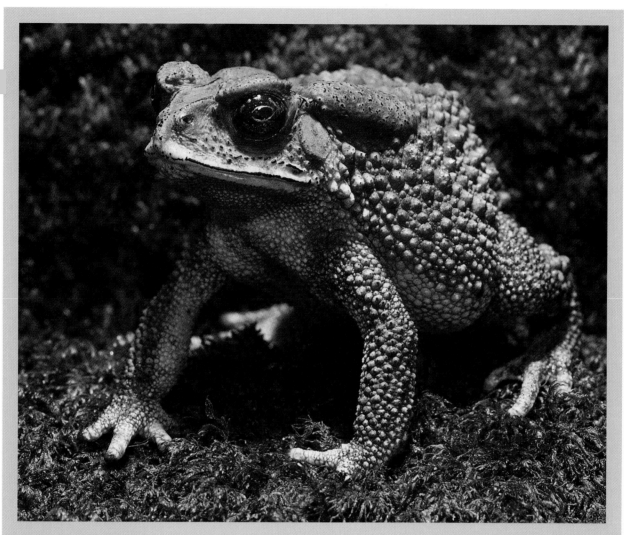

A TOAD TALE

Toads have no luck. First they get blamed for giving people warts (which they can't), then a folk remedy claims you can get rid of warts by rubbing toad urine on them. That's enough to make anyone want to croak. Folk healers must think the pond is a medicine chest: Their strategy for removing warts is to press the fleshy part of a snail on the wart for a few moments. Then your wart will escar*got* away. If you truly want to get rid of warts, don't go to toads or snails. Go to a dermatologist, who will help you deal with the virus that causes this problem.

"Decrease the amount of sugar you take in," says Dr. Kent. "Especially, cut out the alcohol. Historically people complain that when they drink a lot of wine, they get lots of yeast infections." Yeast turns sugar into alcohol, hence the burning in the vagina. But Dr. Kent warns that yeast will even turn sugar substitutes into alcohol.

Also, try to avoid antibiotics, if possible. Many antibiotics kill bacteria that keep yeast in check, so Dr. Kent recommends that if you get an antibiotic prescription, ask your doctor for an additional prescription that will help keep the yeast under control.

A visit to your doctor, who can prescribe an antifungal medication, will also help get rid of your yeast infection. According to Dr. Kent, a yeast infection should clear up within 7 to 14 days.

SEX

Antigens, lymphocytes, T-cells, macrophages—if if you find the immune system's workings puzzling at times, rest assured you're in good company. Some eminently credentialed scientists are every bit as baffled as you are.

Think not? Consider AIDS.

Acquired immune deficiency syndrome: where it came from, where it will go, no one knows. Researchers aren't certain what causes it. Physicians haven't an inkling how to cure it. But one thing is certain: The disease can pulverize a person's immune system.

Not helping efforts to control this epidemic disease is the double whammy AIDS throws at those groping to understand it. For not only does this disease affect the immune system, it also gets passed in bed.

Unlike most of the more than two dozen known sexually transmitted diseases (STDs), however, the AIDS virus is not passed on *solely* in bed; blood transfusions and injections with secondhand needles can also spread the virus. AIDS also differs from other sexually transmitted diseases in that it is presumed lethal, while many others are curable.

One thing STDs share is a common mythology. The old myths went something like this: "You get 'it' from dirty doorknobs . . . from toilet seats . . . from 'bad' girls or boys, never from 'good.'" The new myths sound more sophisticated: "You get 'it' from hot tubs . . . in health clubs . . . from gays, never from 'straights.'"

Let's set the record straight—there's a very good reason why STDs are called STDs. And sex, in all but rare, sad occasions, is a voluntary activity. We choose when, where and with whom we have it. Therefore, STDs are among the most preventable of diseases. All one generally needs is the right kind of information—not myths.

On these pages, we'll throw the bedsheets off seven troublesome myths and get to the naked facts about AIDS and other STDs, and how to prevent them.

MYTH #1: AIDS IS THE MOST COMMON STD

Far from it. AIDS is one of the most recent, the most deadly and the scariest, but it's not the most common STD. That dubious honor would have to go to chlamydia, an affliction that zaps at least four million Americans a year, perhaps many more. "Maybe 10 percent of the population," says Luis de la Maza, M.D., Ph.D., professor of pathology at the University of California, Irvine.

Chlamydia, characterized by redness of and sometimes painful discharge from the penis or vagina, usually passes on its own within two to three weeks. For this reason, it often goes unattended. For women, however, chlamydia can be serious. "It may be the most common cause of infertility in females," says Dr. de la Maza.

MYTH #2: ONLY HOMOSEXUALS AND DRUG USERS CAN GET AIDS

Dead wrong. True, *in the United States,* AIDS is found predominantly among these groups. But in Africa, where AIDS likely originated, this isn't the case. Homosexuality and intravenous drug use are not common in Africa, so heterosexual contact is the primary means of transmission. Although the number of cases among heterosexual nondrug users in the United States is still small, there most definitely have been reported cases of both male-to-female *and* female-to-male transmission of the virus, says Thomas Peterman, M.D., medical epidemiologist with the Division of Sexually Transmitted Diseases at the Centers for Disease Control in Atlanta.

Despite some evidence that heterosexuals are susceptible to the disease, some people just won't believe it. This may be a case of self-imposed ignorance, says Guenter Risse, M.D., Ph.D., chairman of the Department of History of Health Sciences at the University of California, San Francisco. Plagues throughout time have met with myths about how only certain groups could be affected. "If we can create the argument that the victims of a disease

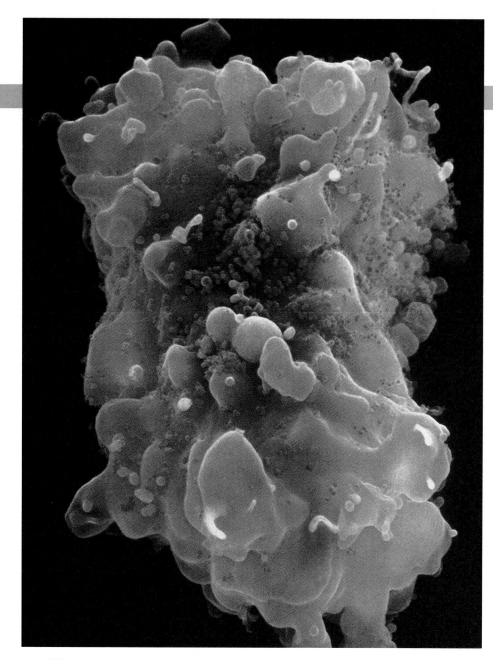

Good guys don't always win. This photo, magnified millions of times, shows the brutal showdown between a helper T-cell and a swarm of AIDS viruses. The outcome is predictable. As the AIDS viruses multiply, they will lay waste to more and more T-cells. Once this key component of the immune system's offensive force is polished off, other body invaders (even the most common and generally harmless bacteria and parasites) are free to run rampant. Eventually, a wearied human host is destroyed from within.

are different from us, maybe not as good as us, then we can pretend that we'll remain disease free," says Dr. Risse.

MYTH #3: HETEROSEXUALS CAN GET AIDS—BUT ONLY THROUGH "ABNORMAL" SEX

Whatever your notion of what constitutes "normal" and "abnormal," it seems that anal sex, because the anal canal is tender and often bleeds during sex, is a favored passageway for the AIDS virus. But what of

conventional intercourse? Experts contend that semen and vaginal secretions are more than enough to carry the virus. Timothy Sankary, M.D., director of the Stop AIDS Foundation of America, says he doubts strongly that all cases of heterosexually transmitted AIDS are caused by knock-down-drag-out sex. And he discounts as "crazy" the notion that unruffled sex is safe-from-AIDS sex. Dr. Sankary maintains that yes, the virus can be passed through conventional intercourse.

But how likely is this to occur? Actually, no

one's sure. One study, reported in the *Journal of the American Medical Association,* found that many women sleep with their AIDS-infected partners hundreds of times without catching the disease. The study also found, however, that one can contract AIDS after only a single encounter—one woman did. Overall, says Dr. Peterman (the study's principal author), sleeping often with an AIDS-infected partner is like playing Russian roulette.

MYTH #4: YOU CAN ALWAYS RECOGNIZE SOMEONE CARRYING THE AIDS VIRUS

You're more apt to recognize someone carrying a picture of Harpo Marx in his wallet. People have been known to harbor the AIDS virus for up to ten years while maintaining an appearance of perfect health and fitness.

If you assume someone carrying the AIDS virus will warn you, consider that the long latency period means many of the infected don't know they're infected. And if you'd expect someone knowingly carrying the virus to tell you, the results of a survey done at the University of California may come as a shock: 12 percent of those surveyed (all homosexual and bisexual men) said that if they found out they had AIDS, they would *not* tell their primary sexual partner, and 27 percent said they would not tell their nonprimary partner.

MYTH #5: IF I USE A CONDOM, I'M SAFE

You're a lot safer than if you don't, but you certainly aren't totally safe. Condoms slip and slide, they break, and in moments of passion they are often forgotten, says Dr. Sankary. In fact, one study found that among condom-using couples in which one partner was infected with AIDS, one in ten of the uninfected spouses became infected within two years—after faithfully using a condom. Further research, says Dr. Sankary, indicates the odds may be even worse.

MYTH #6: GONORRHEA AND SYPHILIS ARE PROBLEMS OF THE PAST

You don't hear as much about them these days, but that's only because AIDS has grabbed the spotlight. Gonorrhea, "the clap," still haunts several million Americans a year.

It's recognized in men by redness at the tip of the penis, a milky discharge and painful urination. Women may also experience painful urination, as well as increased vaginal discharge. In most cases, however, there may be no symptoms at all. But when they do appear, it's typically within two to eight days after infection.

Gonorrhea is usually readily treatable with antibiotics, but doctors are finding that the bacteria are becoming resistant to traditionally prescribed drugs. New strains of antibiotics, however, are being tested all the time.

Not nearly as common as gonorrhea, syphilis still stings several tens of thousands of Americans a year. And for reasons scientists don't fully understand, the incidence of the disease seems to be growing rapidly.

Syphilis is usually signaled by a small, painless sore, or chancre. It starts as a small pimple that gradually enlarges and breaks, forming a small ulcer on the penis, vagina or rectum. This typically happens within one to eight weeks after infection, and the lesion goes away within six weeks, although it often leaves a small scar. At this point, the problem tends to be forgotten, but it's precisely at this point that seeing a doctor becomes urgent, says Mark Martens, M.D., assistant professor at Baylor College of Medicine. If not treated with antibiotics, he says, a rash will likely appear, and the disease can eventually become life-threatening.

MYTH #7: IF I'M GONNA GET IT, I'M GONNA GET IT

D-U-M-B. To be sure, sex is one of the great joys of life, and fear of STDs shouldn't hinder you from participating. But you still should be careful out there.

First (and there's no disagreement among the experts that this goes first): Invest time in getting to know your partner.

Consider *anyone* a potential risk, says Dr. Sankary. "Make sure any new partner has been tested negative *before* you become intimate." AIDS testing is fast, inexpensive and accurate, he says. It does, however, take up to two months after infection for the tests to detect the virus.

So Dr. Sankary advises "a little old-fashioned courtship" for *at least* the first two months of any new relationship. And if the urge should get too strong before that? "Your next choice is a condom," he says. Most experts agree.

Keep in mind, however, that condoms aren't foolproof. If used correctly, however, they will lower your odds of contracting not only AIDS but also gonorrhea, syphilis, chlamydia, herpes and a host of other STDs. For the most protection, choose latex condoms over ones made from animal skin—they're less porous. Make sure the condoms have reservoir tips, so they don't break during ejaculation. Never use petroleum-based lubricants like Vaseline with a latex condom; they can cause it to disintegrate. And if you keep an "emergency" spare in your wallet or purse, remember that latex deteriorates over time.

In addition to condoms and selective sex, Dr. Martens says any of a number of conventional birth control measures—sponges, diaphragms, even the Pill—will somewhat, but not greatly, decrease your chances of contracting an STD. (The importance of washing and urinating after sex, he adds, is largely a myth—these measures probably aren't very helpful.)

Last, don't forget the power of your immune system. A strong immune response offers some protection against STDs, and it is "very important in fighting the recurring diseases like herpes and chlamydia," says Dr. Martens. Anything that depresses your immune system—stress, alcohol, smoking—will allow these diseases to grow."

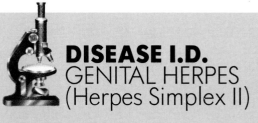

DISEASE I.D.
GENITAL HERPES
(Herpes Simplex II)

DESCRIPTION: Don't let the name fool you—herpes simplex is a pro at complicating lives. Let it into your life and there's no getting it out. Sores in the genital area (sometimes itching or burning), fever and fatigue are the most common things you'll have to live with, on and off. And infection during pregnancy can endanger an unborn child.

INCIDENCE: Herpes is quite common. Some estimates say as many as 20 million Americans may carry the virus. A minority of the infected suffer one to six outbreaks a year.

MODE OF TRANSMISSION: *Sex.* Going to bed with an infected person who shows open sores puts you at almost a 50 percent risk of contracting the disease. You can also get zapped by an infected person without symptoms, but the odds drop to about 1 percent.

DEFENSE FACTORS: Choose your lovers carefully. If you have relations with a person you know is infected, make sure he or she has no sores present—and use a condom.

TREATMENT: If you suspect herpes, see a doctor. Modern medications can't knock out the virus, but they can help you fight off the intermittent attacks. Should you get infected, boost your immune power with proper exercise, sleep, diet and stress management. It won't get rid of the infection but it can do much to help prevent recurrences.

RECOVERY TIME: Without treatment, you may suffer outbreaks that will last from seven to ten days. With treatment, these can be reduced to two to three days. On continuous medication, patients have been known to go two years without an attack.

SMALLPOX

C all it the 10,000-Year War, because that is how long humanity's battle against smallpox has lasted.

It's a war our immune system eventually won—with a little help from modern medicine. But we paid an enormous price along the way: the lives of millions of mothers and fathers and sons and daughters, all taken by a disease that began killing us deep in the night of our most ancient history.

"It's so hard for people today to comprehend just how feared this disease was," says D. A. Henderson, M.D., the epidemiologist who led the World Health Organization (WHO) campaign against smallpox.

"People were totally and absolutely terrified of it, and with good reason. *Variola major*, the more lethal form of the disease, killed 20 to 40 percent of its victims. Most of those who survived were permanently scarred and some were blinded. "No other infection even comes close" in terms of devastation.

No wonder governments took smallpox very seriously. Even after the disease was on the wane, some kept enormous, empty hospitals ready just in case the virus resurfaced.

"England, for example, kept *six* hospitals on standby," Dr. Henderson says, "and the country was smallpox-free at the time."

But when you look at the numbers involved, such caution becomes instantly understandable. Even as late as 1967, the virus *killed* two million people, blinded a few hundred thousand more and scarred no one knows how many additional thousands. The estimated cost to the world—a billion dollars annually.

FROM PHARAOH TO FADEOUT

The disease was on the march at least 3,000 years ago—when Pharaoh Ramses V died of a severe infection that was probably smallpox. But scientists speculate that the very first case may have developed *10,000* years ago, in a farmer targeted by a mutant animal pox virus.

The traditional pattern: infection by inhaled virus, high fever and muscle pain after 10 to 12 days,

and then the characteristic two-week-long rash—small blisters covering the entire body but thickest on face, arms and legs.

But that pattern is now history. Although vaccines had been in use since the 18th century, it wasn't until 1967, when WHO launched an intensified worldwide campaign, that the chain of transmission was broken.

On May 8, 1980—more than two years after the last known case—WHO made the official announcement that "The world and all its people have won freedom from smallpox."

But how could we be so sure? Dr. Henderson says—with a small smile—that they learned from experience.

"Over the years, we found that in every instance where smallpox reappeared in an area where we thought we'd eradicated it—and this included the most primitive of rural areas—it did so within eight months. If we didn't see another case within eight months, the disease just wasn't there anymore."

WHO kept searching diligently for cases, waiting three times longer than that eight-month period to give itself a safety margin before declaring the virus extinct. So when it did make the announcement, it was sure about it.

The result?

Every year that the world is free of smallpox, $2 billion and two million lives will be saved.

"The only place you'll find smallpox in the world today is in glass vials, frozen inside laboratory refrigerators," Dr. Henderson says.

And no, a burglar with a crowbar isn't likely to accidentally reinfect the world: The laboratories holding the virus just happen to be two of the most secure on earth—the Centers for Disease Control in Atlanta and the Research Institute for Viral Preparations in Moscow.

In the last days of the war against smallpox, cash rewards like the one offered in this poster proved very effective in bringing to light cases that otherwise might have been missed.

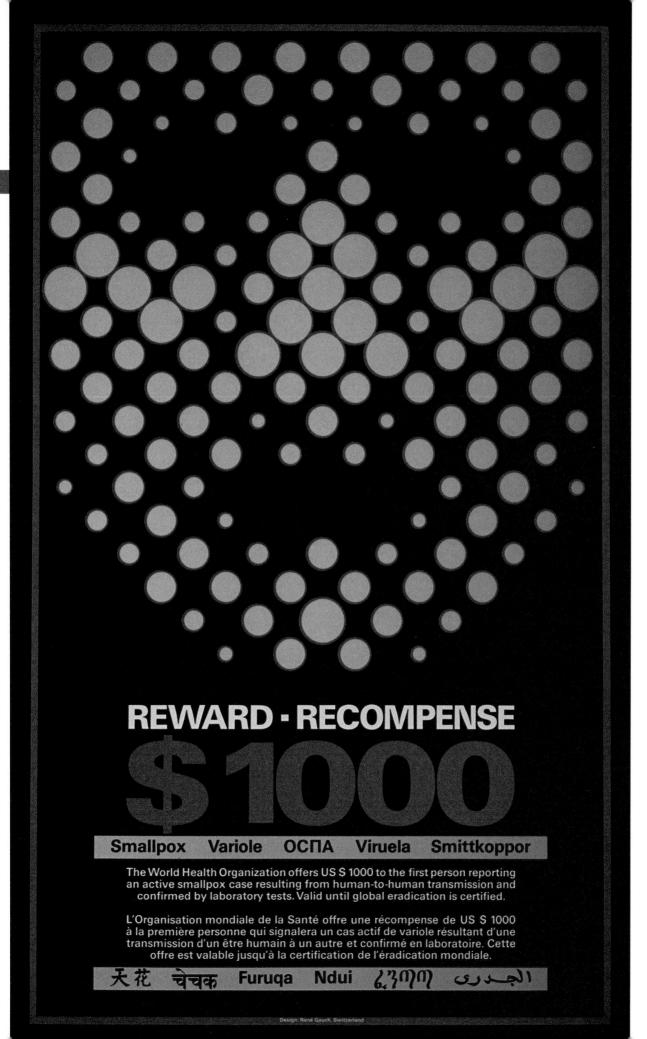

REWARD · RECOMPENSE

$1000

Smallpox   Variole   ОСПА   Viruela   Smittkoppor

The World Health Organization offers US $ 1000 to the first person reporting an active smallpox case resulting from human-to-human transmission and confirmed by laboratory tests. Valid until global eradication is certified.

L'Organisation mondiale de la Santé offre une récompense de US $ 1000 à la première personne qui signalera un cas actif de variole résultant d'une transmission d'un être humain à un autre et confirmé en laboratoire. Cette offre est valable jusqu'à la certification de l'éradication mondiale.

天花　चेचक　**Furuqa　Ndui**　ረጉጦ　الجدرى

Design: René Gauch, Switzerland

SMOKING

U nless you decided a couple of decades ago that no news is good news—that your unplugged television set makes for an attractive plant stand and your unread newspapers provide ideal all-weather insulation—you've certainly heard the word: Cigarette smoking is bad for your health. In fact, it's an absolute disaster.

"Cigarette smoking has been identified as the single most important source of preventable morbidity [illness] and premature mortality [death] in each of the reports of the U.S. Surgeon General produced since 1964," notes the *New England Journal of Medicine*. A partial list of problems linked to lighting up includes heart attacks, strokes and other forms of coronary heart disease; lung cancer and cancers of the larynx, bladder and pancreas; gastrointestinal disease; and diseases of the mouth.

Scientists have conducted thousands of studies to smoke out the connections between disease and the tar, nicotine and other toxic substances present in cigarettes. They have also been taking a microscopically close look at how tobacco smoke causes changes in the immune system, changes which could account for lowered resistance to disease.

Researchers have found, for example, that smokers have an impaired ability to produce antibodies to fight infection to their upper respiratory tracts. And that their T-cells—immune cells that regulate the response to infection—are less active.

But perhaps the most promising discovery that immune researchers have made in assembling their case against smoking is this finding from the University of Minnesota School of Public Health: Smokers produce large numbers of white blood cells, especially neutrophils—white cells that normally seize and swallow enemy cells—but these white blood cells can't get the job done. This condition occurs after smoking just a few cigarettes. And scientists

LEUKOCYTES ON THE MARCH

Leukocytes, a type of infection-fighting white blood cell, increase abnormally among smokers, says a study of more than 62,000 adults. The more cigarettes people smoke each day, the higher their leukocyte counts rise. Scientists theorize that excess leukocytes contribute to heart disease rather than deter it. These levels decline gradually when smokers quit.

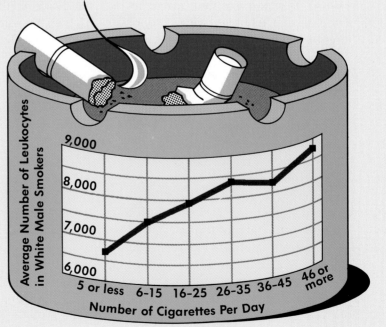

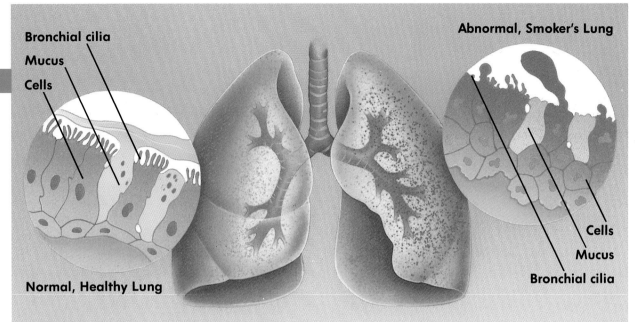

Bronchial cilia

Mucus

Cells

Abnormal, Smoker's Lung

Cells

Mucus

Bronchial cilia

Normal, Healthy Lung

CIGARETTES CRIPPLE CILIA

Bronchial cilia, microscopic hairlike structures that defend the lungs against invasions by foreign particles, are immobilized by cigarette smoking. Cilia in a healthy nonsmoker's lung (left) efficiently sweep away a thin layer of particle-packed mucus. The cilia of a smoker (right) are weak, which allows mucus to build up and results in the familiar "smoker's cough."

believe it may be linked to arteriosclerosis—a disease (common among smokers) in which the heart's arteries thicken and lose their efficiency.

"My guess is that the high white blood cell count precedes coronary heart disease, that it somehow *causes* the arteriosclerosis process," says Richard Grimm, M.D., associate professor of epidemiology and researcher in the Minnesota study.

How do the extra white blood cells cause heart disease? One theory is that leukocytes, a particular kind of white blood cell, cluster around weak sections of the blood vessels and release free radicals. "These are highly unstable compounds that may damage the inner lining of blood vessels," Dr. Grimm explains.

Other theories are that proliferating leukocytes plug up blood vessels temporarily or permanently, that they flow in an abnormal fashion through blood vessels and gang up in certain areas or that they cause the vessels to swell.

Cigarettes may be murderous when it comes to immune responses to cancer, too.

"We know that smoking is the single most impor-

tant factor causing lung cancer. The data is irrefutable," says Barbara Phillips, M.D., professor of pulmonary medicine at the University of Kentucky Medical Center. "In studying the mechanism for this, we've now found that smoking suppresses natural killer cell activity. These are the cells whose job it is to seek out and destroy cancer cells before they gain a foothold."

Dr. Phillips conducted a study that showed that the killer cells of both heavy smokers and lung cancer patients were less effective than normal when it came to destroying cancer cells.

Ex-smokers may breathe easier to learn that their high white blood cell counts decline and natural killer cell activity perks up once they kick the habit. In fact, their immune system functions overall get back on track.

Some people quit cold turkey; others find hypnosis or nicotine gum helpful. Programs that provide continued support by a physician or a group are most effective, says Dr. Phillips. As difficult as putting cigarettes down can be, it's just the pick-me-up a smoker's immune system needs.

TRAVEL

You are deep in the heart of a Moroccan bazaar, surrounded by women in veils and men with huge knives. Camels belch, dogs bark, and over it all a hot sun burns brightly.

You almost stagger with relief when a local vendor thrusts a cup of ice and a bottle of cola into your hand. A coin goes into his outstretched palm one moment, the soda and half the ice down your throat the next.

Cool, cold, blessed relief—and a sure-fire prescription for misery. In this case, it's not the soft drink or the cup or something on the vendor's hands that's to blame for this clear case of turista, a malady also known as traveler's diarrhea. It's the ice.

"Traveler's diarrhea is the single biggest health threat most people will encounter when traveling in developing countries," says James Wilkerson, M.D., an inveterate rolling stone who is the author of *Medicine for Mountaineering.*

"It's caused either by a virus or bacteria, but both almost always are the result of fecal contamination of the water supply. And water is a notorious source of infection."

But not the only one. The food you eat—mainly raw vegetables and fruit—is another source. (Cooked foods are usually not the problem, because the heat kills the bugs.)

According to Dr. Wilkerson, people using the local streams and rivers for things besides bathing are almost always to blame for the contaminated water supply. And crops are often tainted because human waste is a popular fertilizer in many regions.

"Sanitation is something that's very poorly understood in large parts of the world outside of Western Europe and North America," Dr. Wilkerson says. "I recall seeing a man brushing his teeth in river water downstream from someone else washing his clothes, both downstream from a large village—and another guy farther upstream urinating in it."

The bug that's most often responsible for getting a stranglehold on your gut is a species of bacteria called *Escherichia coli*—*E. coli* for short. And while it's true that a Spaniard visiting New York can get the infection as easily as an American visiting Uganda, the Spaniard is less likely to get it simply because U.S. water is rarely contaminated with fecal material.

"*E. coli* is an organism we all carry in our intestinal system," Dr. Wilkerson continues. "It produces mild toxins that, over time, we usually develop immunity to. What happens when you travel is that you eat

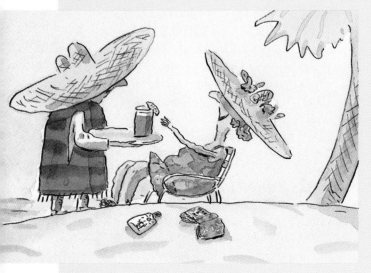

SAFETY SPANISH

Installing the following phrases in your memory bank can help make dining out a less traumatic experience—and turista someone else's problem—the next time you're in a Spanish-speaking country.

1. Is this juice freshly squeezed? *Este jugo, es recien hecho?*
2. Has water been added to it? *Se le agrego agua?*
3. Please give me an unopened bottle of plain water. *Por favor deme una botella cerrada de agua.*
4. Please boil the water for at least ten minutes. *Por favor, hierva el agua por lo menos diez minutos.*
5. Is it pasteurized? *Es pastuerizado?*

or drink a new variety, producing a slightly different toxin—one your body can't neutralize—and you end up with diarrhea."

Which explains why the locals in some of the more exotic locales that attract Americans can tolerate the food and water while you can't. But you *could* if you were willing to acclimate by suffering through a bout of turista.

GETTING BACK ALIVE

But you don't want to *live* there; you just want to visit. And you want it to be a pleasant visit.

A few simple precautions will go a long way toward making your exotic vacation a healthy and relaxing romp in the sun—not the emergency room. Here are Dr. Wilkerson's recommendations.

Stay away from local water. "Don't *ever* drink the water," Dr. Wilkerson says. "I don't care where you are, at your hotel or down in the embassy—don't drink the water."

Bottled water is almost always safe, and it is a good solution for brushing your teeth and washing your hands. If you have to drink suspect H_2O or use it for personal hygiene, disinfect it first—either with iodine, using the method described in the box "New Ways to Make Your Water Safe" on page 102, or with iodine tablets such as Potable Aqua. Caution: Make sure the tablets are fresh, since pills in an open bottle can lose almost half their iodine in a single week.

"I practically disinfect the water I wash my *feet* in," Dr. Wilkerson laughs.

Eat only well-cooked foods and peeled fruits. "Years ago, they used to soak things like salad and vegetables in a solution of potassium permanganate, but it just didn't work," Dr. Wilkerson says. "The only reliable safeguards—given the reality that in most cases you have absolutely no control over how your food's being prepared or the conditions under which it's being prepared—are to stick with well-cooked food. Don't eat salads or raw vegetables of any kind and eat only fruit you've peeled yourself. Everything else is off-limits."

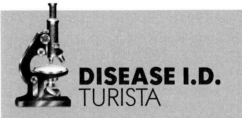

DISEASE I.D.
TURISTA

DESCRIPTION: Traveler's diarrhea—*turista* in Spanish, from the language spoken in countries where lots of Americans get it—is simply diarrhea that develops while people are traveling. It is characterized by loose, watery stools, abdominal cramps and occasionally chills and sweating—just the things that can spoil a vacation.

INCIDENCE: Endemic, occurring wherever people travel, although it's most prevalent in developing countries, and affecting almost everyone who travels.

MODES OF TRANSMISSION: Bacteria, viruses or protozoa that are known to invade raw food and water. Ingestion of the causative organisms via contaminated utensils, hands, food and water.

DEFENSE FACTORS: Disinfection of *all* tap or river water used for drinking or brushing the teeth, or use of clean bottled water; basic cleanliness; and limiting meals to well-cooked foods, peeled vegetables and fruits. Avoid all raw vegetables, salads and unpeeled fruits. Eat only foods that are served hot and drink only beverages that have been bottled.

TREATMENT: Rest and more rest. Antibiotics may be indicated in severe cases. Sometimes antimotility agents are necessary. Fluids are important to prevent dehydration.

RECOVERY TIME: Most of the afflicted will be fully recovered within three or four days.

What about things like ice cream? Or candy bars? Dr. Wilkerson says it depends. "Candy bars are probably fine, assuming we're talking about the professionally packaged and manufactured kind like the brands you find back home. But ice cream is out. I had some climbers in Kathmandu, the capital city in Nepal, leave the hotel and grab some sherbet at an American-based chain. They almost died."

Watch your personal hygiene. "Wash your hands before you eat—and be religious about it," Dr. Wilkerson says. "You can infect yourself just as easily by ignoring basic hygiene as you can by drinking the local water."

WHEN ALL ELSE FAILS
But what do you do if it all goes wrong? If a bacterium somehow punctures your armor anyway? Well,

take heart. In most cases there's very little need to do anything at all.

"Usually, people are going to get better on their own in two or three days," Dr. Wilkerson says. "And that's usually what I recommend—let the disease run its course. There's some solid evidence that treating with something like Lomotil—which certainly works, by the way—may in fact prolong the course of the infection by blocking the body's efforts to flush the bacteria out of the intestines. I usually prescribe just rest, lots of fluids and more rest."

If you're at special risk for serious complications —as someone suffering from inflammatory bowel disease would be—you may want to ask your physician to prescribe Bactrim or Septra, antimicrobial drugs proven effective in preventing the onset of traveler's diarrhea. But for the average, healthy traveler,

A CASE OF CABIN FEVER

Can the confined cabin space and shared air on an airplane increase your risk of health problems? There's a good chance the answer may be yes: 72 percent of the passengers aboard a plane stalled for 3 hours by engine trouble in Alaska came down with influenza within three

days of the incident. The fact that everyone aboard was going to the same small town made the study possible—and led scientists to speculate that "similar outbreaks could result from crowded flights with an infectious person and not be documented or noticed."

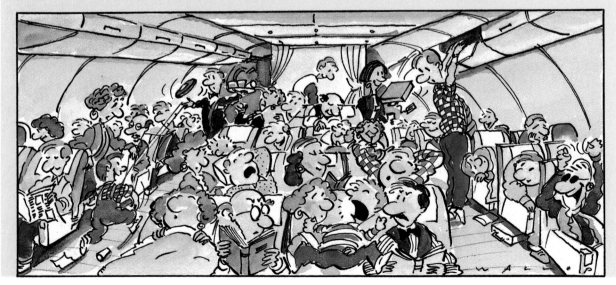

Dr. Wilkerson recommends against routine use of antibiotics as a preventive.

"One, you always have the possibility of an allergic reaction to the drug," he says. "People do die from sensitivities to antibiotics. And two, it's an expensive option that can present other problems. People tend to get careless about what they eat and how they eat it, and there are worse bugs out there than *E. coli* that can use that opportunity to come on board."

But there's a safe, nonmedical option open to those who prefer to avoid antibiotics or simply choose not to spend the money. Pepto-Bismol, for reasons that aren't precisely clear, is also very effective at preventing turista. The only drawback—you have to drink a bottle a day, which adds up to an awful lot of pink glassware in your luggage.

THE HEAVY HITTERS

If a particularly nasty case of diarrhea doesn't show any improvement after a few days, it's wise to see a doctor.

Though the chances are remote, what you think is a nasty touch of turista may actually be something with teeth and claws—cholera, for example, or typhoid.

"Cholera is still a major health threat in many parts of the world, and you can't assume you're protected just because you've been vaccinated against it," Dr. Wilkerson says.

"The vaccines for cholera and typhoid are both bacterial vaccines, which characteristically aren't as effective as viral versions. If you've been vaccinated, you probably won't get quite as sick. But remember, cholera and typhoid can kill people. You can still get really ill."

Cholera and typhoid both cause severe, life-threatening diarrhea. In certain regions, however, risk is unusually high: Diarrheal disease is the leading killer in Nepal, Dr. Wilkerson says.

But if you do get it, don't panic: Medical care is necessary, but staying alive is chiefly a matter of keeping your fluid intake high until the disease runs its course.

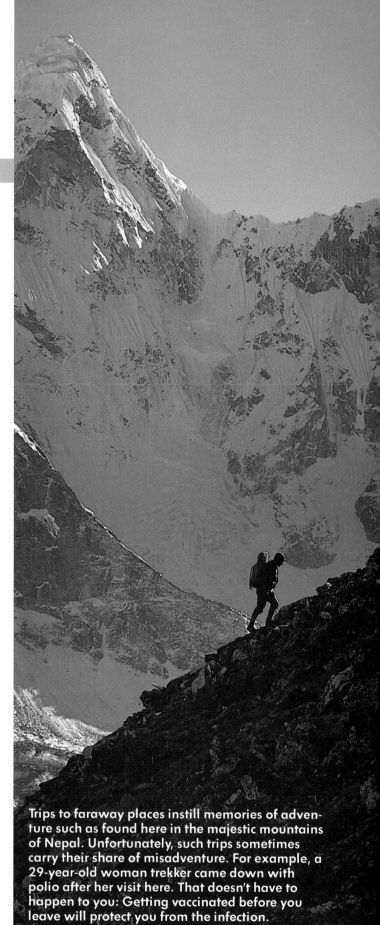

Trips to faraway places instill memories of adventure such as found here in the majestic mountains of Nepal. Unfortunately, such trips sometimes carry their share of misadventure. For example, a 29-year-old woman trekker came down with polio after her visit here. That doesn't have to happen to you: Getting vaccinated before you leave will protect you from the infection.

WEATHER

Olduvai Gorge, Africa—1,000,000 B.C. Thunder rumbles. Lightning crackles on the horizon. And a steady hard rain pelts at the red stone rim of the gorge. On a ledge below, beneath an overhang, a prehistoric man lifts his head to look at the sky, eyes dàrk beneath eyebrows dripping with rainwater. Thunder booms in the distance, and in response, he shakes his fist.

New York, New York—Today. Snow frosts the concrete canyons of Manhattan. A pale winter sun throws mother-of-pearl highlights on an otherwise gray sky. And cold winds off the Hudson hurl sheets of icy water over the breakwaters. A man on the sidewalk curses when a passing cab splash-paints his expensive trenchcoat with gallons of gutter wash. He shakes a fist at the dented yellow shape retreating into the distant murk.

Yes, it's cold outside! Winter weather and all its ramifications—like an unexpected snowfall—have been known to help compromise a strong immune system. But there are ways to fight back. Getting out in the sunshine and doing something active is helpful in fighting the wintertime blues.

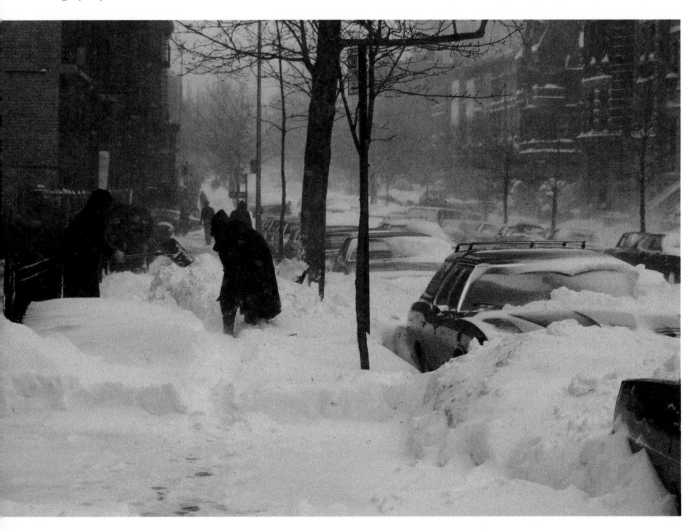

An ancient indignity and a modern inconvenience, weather is something we've been complaining about since the first of humanity's simian ancestors left the trees to walk the prairies.

But a threat to our health? Something that can almost literally rip the vigor out of our immune systems?

That's a fact, states Laurentian University neuroscience professor Michael A. Persinger, Ph.D., author of *The Weather Matrix and Human Behavior.*

"Whenever you look at the relationship between weather and immune function, the first thing you have to be aware of is that you're looking at a matrix—a complex of factors," says Dr. Persinger. "They're all so closely related you can't point to just one and say it's responsible for a particular change in the immune system.

"But I'm convinced that weather in the larger sense of the word has a major effect on our immunocapacity, our resistance to infection."

It's a conviction that lends real credence to the old saying "feeling under the weather."

A CLOUDY DAY IN YOUR BRAIN

Just how does the weather manage to get you down? The precise mechanisms haven't been identified, but the immune-system component responsible has been confirmed with reasonable certainty: It starts in the brain, or more precisely, the amygdala and hippocampus portions of the brain.

"There's no doubt that the hypothalamus is the ultimate controller of the immune system, but the amygdala, with the adjacent hippocampus, is the modulator, or fine tuner," Dr. Persinger says. "This is the structure we think regulates the interaction between weather and the immune system."

But according to Dr. Persinger, it's more a question of *when* weather affects our immunity than of *how.* Day-to-day weather—a sunny spell here, some passing showers there—really doesn't do much to us. But take a particular weather "matrix"—heat, high humidity and stagnant air, for example, or cold

plus ultra-low humidity and high winds—and the impact can be significant. A classic example: seasonal affective disorder, or SAD, a syndrome that sinks its victims into the doldrums, causing depression, fatigue and sleepiness. Scientists believe it's directly related to the decrease of sunlight in the wintertime.

Because SAD affects so many people, it offers researchers an important window into nuances of immune-system functioning, says Dr. Persinger. "In this instance, we know that during the winter months the synthesis of melatonin [a brain regulatory chemical] increases markedly, apparently in direct correlation with the decrease in available light."

The result? Sleep problems, depression—and a drop in immune function.

THE WINTER OF OUR DISCONTENT

So while you're looking forward to summer—hoping your mood will improve with the weather—keep this in mind: Winter is indeed the season most likely to make your immune system shiver.

"That's a correct statement for a number of reasons," Dr. Persinger says. "The cold can directly suppress your immune system, for example, but it has other consequences bearing on your health as well."

Consider that you're inside almost all the time and that there are fewer interesting things to do in the winter unless you're a skiing enthusiast. That means you're probably feeling bored, because there's nothing to do. Because you're bored and not doing anything, you get depressed. Because you're depressed, your immune system starts to wobble. Because you're inside, you're exposed to much higher concentrations of disease "vectors"—primarily germs and viruses from other people. Your already trembling immune system finds it can't cope with one of them, and *wham*—you're sick.

So the next time someone kids you about your winter vacation in Mexico, just smile and tell them you're actually going to Acapulco to work on your tan *and* your immune system.

XENOBIOTIC INFECTIONS

The world wanted to give them a ticker-tape parade. Instead, they were slapped into the isolation of strict quarantine. Even President Nixon had to content himself with viewing the Apollo 11 astronauts through glass.

The year was 1969. Astronauts Neil Armstrong, Buzz Aldrin and Mike Collins had just come back from the first trip to the moon, and the President of the United States was forbidden to shake their hands. It wouldn't do for the commander-in-chief to be exposed to a close encounter of the infectious kind.

Germs in space? Extraterrestrial microbes? Xenobiotic (*xeno* means foreign and *biotic* means life) infection? Is *that* why they locked up the astronauts?

Space is the final frontier. And when humans decide to boldly go where no one has gone before, they risk coming in contact with what no one's immune system has ever dealt with before.

Scientists from the National Aeronautics and Space Administration (NASA) weren't about to test whether the human immune system is capable of meeting such a challenge.

ARE MICROINVADERS A THREAT?

"If a microbe *did* come back from the moon, it would be in an alien environment on earth and would be killed off very quickly, in my opinion," says Lawrence Dietlein, M.D., Ph.D., assistant director for life sciences at NASA's Johnson Space Center in Houston. "But some scientists thought that the earth with all its great nutrients and oxygen might be just the perfect incubator for some strange form of life that might be on the lunar surface."

Dr. Dietlein remembers the extensive planning and precautions involved in welcoming back the earth's first lunar visitors.

When the Apollo 11 capsule splashed down in the Pacific Ocean, frogmen swabbed down the exterior of the spacecraft with Betadine, an iodine disinfectant. Then they popped open the hatch of the capsule and tossed in special "biological isolation garments." The astronauts, who had worn special spacesuits during their stay on the moon, had to don equally special suits for their terrestrial return. The suits' respirators were filtered to prevent the escape of any germs the astronauts might have picked up during their voyage.

The space travelers then stepped into a raft filled with disinfectant and were hoisted to a quarantine van on board the U.S.S. Hornet. The trailerlike van served to transport them to the specially built, multimillion-dollar Lunar Receiving Laboratory in Houston. The space crew's quarantine lasted almost three weeks before they were released to bask in the adulation of the nation.

Rock and soil samples from the moon were handled with equal caution. After weeks of careful study, exposing numerous species of plants and animals to lunar samples, scientists found . . . nothing. No bugs. No germs. Nothing to be concerned about. And that didn't surprise anybody, either.

So why the fuss?

The immune system develops defenses against known germs, but new challenges can be serious. Witness what happened to American Indians when they encountered smallpox for the first time. The lethal disease wiped out whole tribes.

"We were also addressing the concerns of the farmer who was worried that some virulent organism from space would destroy his cotton or his corn or his hogs," says microbiologist Adrian Mandel, Ph.D., with the Ames Research Center in Moffit Field, California. Dr. Mandel was on the Interagency Committee on Back Contamination that advised NASA how to handle the returning astronauts and their cargo.

TAKE ME TO YOUR LEADER

Other scientists take a friendlier view toward microbes from space. If astronauts do encounter a new microbe and bring it back from the moon or elsewhere, scientists' first concern should be to keep it alive so they can study it, says Thomas Jukes, Ph.D., professor of biophysics at the University of California in Berkeley. He finds it highly unlikely that such a microbe could pose a threat.

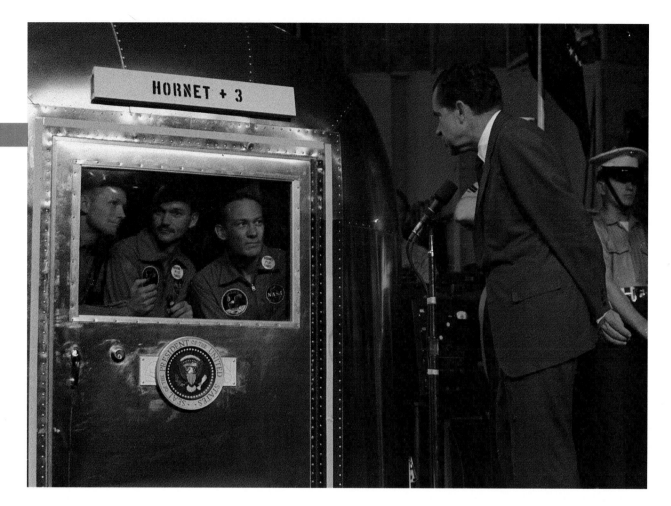

"Pathogenic organisms have evolved over millions of years by accommodating themselves to their host," says Dr. Jukes. Smallpox virus is harmful to humans, for example, because it evolved with humans.

Since diseases are very "species specific"—humans and animals often can't catch each other's diseases—there's little reason to assume that microbes from the realm of the Purple People Eater would be lethal to Homo sapiens.

A number of researchers suggest that politics rather than science was the real reason for extensive quarantine precautions following the lunar landings. NASA's Dr. Dietlein believes the precautions were in part to reassure a nation raised on sci-fi visions of monsters and blobs. It wouldn't do to panic the masses.

THE RED PLANET WAITS

And yet . . . and yet . . . there is that little edge of concern that creeps into even the most scientific discussions.

"Even as I talk to you, I could be wrong," says Dr. Mandel. "There could be something unknown,

President Nixon delivers his welcoming address to Apollo 11 astronauts Neil Armstrong, Mike Collins and Buzz Aldrin, who are confined in a quarantine van aboard the U.S.S. Hornet. Only after weeks of careful study were researchers sure that microscopic space invaders hadn't accompanied the crew home from humankind's first trip to the moon.

unexplained, a first-time occurrence."

And so history seems destined to repeat itself. The concerns are the same, the politics haven't gone away, and the red planet looms on the horizon.

Scientists working on planning expeditions to Mars are considering the possibility of quarantining soil and rock samples on an orbiting space station before bringing them back to earth, says Michael B. Duke, Ph.D., chief of solar system exploration at NASA's Johnson Space Center.

"The environment of Mars is not conducive to life forms as we know them," he says. "However, a space station 'quarantine' would be a logical way to both study the samples and protect the environment on earth."

157

40 WORST INFECTIONS

Good health is the result of an endless battle, the consequence of slaughter on a grand scale—namely, the bugs your immune system mangles by the million each and every day.

It's reassuring to know that the enemy usually loses, but there's a hard core of hostiles out there, a rogues' gallery if you will, that occasionally penetrates our living shield.

Usually, it doesn't matter. The bad guys may catch up with the wagon train, but they can't make it stop—most of the time. Occasionally, though, a few tough ones pull it off. They can be thought of as the infectious felons in the ongoing drama of the immune system.

Who's who on the Most-Feared Infectious Felons List? Following you'll find the 40 most persistent of these health burglars, according to medical research and drawing on statistics provided by the Centers for Disease Control (CDC). Within the six groups, infections are ranked roughly in order of severity and incidence, with the most severe and/or most common listed first in each category.

The medical explanation for each is based upon information provided by Harvey Friedman, M.D., associate professor of medicine, Division of Infectious Diseases, University of Pennsylvania School of Medicine.

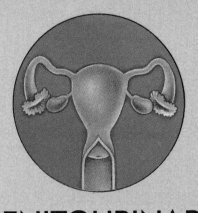

GENITOURINARY INFECTIONS

(SEXUALLY TRANSMITTED DISEASES)

ACQUIRED IMMUNE DEFICIENCY SYNDROME (AIDS)

AIDS may or may not have been brought to the United States by Gaetan Dugas—the notoriously promiscuous Canadian airline steward who is thought by many to have played a major role in establishing AIDS in this country in the late 1970s and early 1980s. Dugas, who may have acquired AIDS on a trip to the Caribbean, was linked to so many early victims of the disease that researchers nicknamed him Patient Zero—the one who started the American epidemic.

But this deadly disease is here in such force that who brought it probably doesn't matter. By 1988, more than 50,000 cases had been reported to the CDC.

The virus that causes AIDS is transmitted via exchange of bodily fluids—most often through sexual contact, sharing needles (a risk for drug abusers) or exposure (usually during hospitalization) to contaminated blood. AIDS is such a threatening disease because it impairs certain immune functions so drastically that infections we could normally shrug off turn vicious and kill.

"There's a gradual decline over a period of years in the ability of an infected person's immune system to fight infection," Dr. Friedman says. "Toward the end, deterioration accelerates rapidly. Patients come down with frequent and often fatal opportunistic infections—infections that normally don't cause serious disease in a healthy person. And they often develop tumors, which are the second most common cause of death in AIDS patients."

Unfortunately, although the medical community knows what the virus does, it still isn't sure how it does it. A cure is not yet available.

"The basic message is clear—your only option is to try and prevent it," Dr. Friedman says. "And AIDS *is* a preventable disease, one you can avoid by modifying your sexual behavior."

Medical care for people who already have the disease is limited to treating the infections they develop and providing general support. But powerful antiviral drugs like zidovudine (Retrovir)—which act by interfering with the virus's ability to reproduce itself—have been found to extend life by as much as six months to a year in many cases.

SYPHILIS

It killed Chicago gangster Al Capone, but syphilis used to be better known as a sailor's disease—a penalty for taking "a girl in every port" too seriously.

It continues to penalize people today: Syphilis afflicted more than 35,000 Americans in a recent year.

Symptoms produced by this bacteria include an initial painless sore or ulcer that appears in the genital area 10 to 40 days after infection. If left untreated, the disease eventually permeates the body, damaging skin, bones, joints, heart, lungs, blood vessels and the brain.

Treatment is simple, however: Penicillin puts a permanent stop to syphilis.

GONORRHEA

Unlike syphilis, which can proceed undetected for many years, gonorrhea's presence is painfully obvious, at least in men: It produces inflammation of the urethra, pain, and often a purulent discharge. Infected women may notice a discharge but often acquire the disease without noticeable symptoms.

Gonorrhea is the most common sexually transmitted disease—800,000-plus cases were reported to the CDC in a recent year. And—big surprise—it's caused by bacteria that can only be passed from one person to another during sex.

That's *how* you get it. What to do about this bacterial infection after you get it isn't so obvious.

"Gonorrhea has become much more difficult to treat in the last decade, with the development of strains that are strongly resistant to penicillin," Dr. Friedman says.

"Acceptable treatment today is essentially ceftriaxone, which most strains still respond to, with the addition of tetracycline to handle other infections that may mimic gonorrhea," he says.

GENITAL HERPES

Crossing your legs is the last thing you want to do if you've got this sexually transmitted version of the herpes simplex virus. Painful blister clusters in the groin area, occasionally accompanied by painful genital ulcers, can make life miserable. Like gonorrhea, genital herpes affects large numbers of people—in a recent year, an estimated 450,000 men and women sought their physicians' advice on how to cope with the infection.

The bad news: There's no cure. "Once you have the infection, it tends to recur periodically for years—it's not a one-time thing," Dr. Friedman says.

The good news: Treatment with appropriate antiviral drugs like acyclovir (Zovirax) can markedly shorten the course of the initial outbreak, which is usually the longest—up to three weeks—and the worst.

More good news: "It's not a very infectious virus, despite what you may have heard," Dr. Friedman says. "You really have to rub it in, à la sexual intercourse."

Getting it from a toilet seat? "Well, that's not impossible, but it is highly unlikely," he says.

NONSPECIFIC URETHRITIS (NSU)

When you try to go the bathroom and nothing happens except *hurt,* this is a likely villain.

Urethritis refers to inflammation of the urethra—the tube that carries urine from your bladder to the outside world. It can be caused by any number of organisms, but most often by one in particular.

"Nonspecific urethritis is really chlamydia," Dr.

Friedman says. "There are a few other agents that can cause it, but most patients with NSU have chlamydia."

Technically, this organism is a cross of sorts between a bacterium and a virus, sharing some characteristics of both. Chlamydia produces symptoms very similar to those of gonorrhea—including pain and discharge—and is often confused with it.

"A major advantage of using tetracyline to treat gonorrhea is the cross-over effect: It's also effective against chlamydia," Dr. Friedman says. "If there's even a hint of a doubt about the diagnosis as gonorrhea, tetracyline is the drug of choice."

VAGINITIS

You probably realize that *itis* means inflammation of something. Vaginitis means inflammation of the vaginal canal, from any cause. It's typically accompanied by pain and a purulent discharge.

"That's the real issue with vaginitis—it has many, many causes," Dr. Friedman emphasizes. If herpes, gonorrhea or chlamydia isn't to blame, the next most common cause is *gardnerella vaginalis*, a bacterial infection.

"The key to making the diagnosis here is the discharge," Dr. Friedman says. "Gardnerella often has a distinctly unpleasant odor, which the others don't. The best treatment is a drug called metronidazole (Flagyl)."

Candida, a fungus, is another common cause of vaginitis. *Candida* typically produces a thick, white, odorless discharge. Treatment most often is with a drug called clotrimazole.

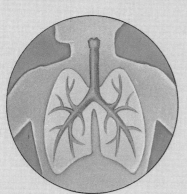

RESPIRATORY INFECTIONS

PNEUMONIA

You can think of this as a supremely bad chest cold: Your lungs are on fire with inflammation and you can't get enough air—fluid released by the angry tissue is blocking the free flow of oxygen.

"Pneumonia just means an infection of the lung, and there are many, many different causes: many different viruses, many different bacteria. But bacteria are the leading cause," Dr. Friedman says.

The bacterium most often responsible for lung infections that develop at home is the pneumococcus. But if you come down with inflamed lungs in the hospital, any one of a small army of organisms could be the culprit.

One of the leading bacterial contenders is *Klebsiella pneumoniae*. "This is a fairly common cause in severely ill patients," Dr. Friedman says.

Other common offenders include *Staphylococcus aureus* and *Streptococcus pneumoniae*—the latter bug may periodically turn your throat into a pain generator.

"We'll usually treat outpatient pneumonia with erythromycin," says Dr. Friedman, "but the hospitalized patient will get a much broader treatment—possibly several antibiotics simultaneously, until we get the cultures back from the lab and know exactly which organism we're dealing with."

INFLUENZA

The flu has been known to be a major killer—an epidemic in 1918 took more lives than World War I—but today it's seldom more than an inconvenient misery for most of us. And because there are so many different and constantly mutating strains out there, you could get it ten times in a row without catching the same strain twice.

The flu is a major cause of pneumonia, too, but with one important difference: This is a viral infection, which makes the pneumonia it may produce more difficult to combat than bacterially produced varieties.

"An essential difference between bacterial and viral infections is that bacteria are self-contained, independent," Dr. Friedman says. "We can attack them with antibiotics that act directly on the individual organisms. Viruses rely on the machinery of a host cell to replicate themselves. Attacking them is much more difficult since they're actually inside our own cells: We have to somehow damage the virus *without* injuring the cell."

Vaccines can markedly reduce the severity of the infection, but they won't necessarily prevent it. And because the virus mutates so frequently, vaccines have to be updated and replaced with each new epidemic.

Those epidemics usually occur about midwinter. "Why that happens isn't well understood," says Dr. Friedman, "but the virus clearly has a cycle, and that cycle appears to be related to climate."

Influenza chiefly affects the upper airway—your nose and throat. It is dangerous chiefly to the very young and very old. Senior citizens at special risk are frequently vaccinated on their physician's advice. But for most of us for whom the flu is not a life-threatening disease, treatment consists chiefly of rest, fluids and medication to relieve symptoms.

"A drug called amantadine is available now that helps significantly if it's given within the first 48 hours. It interferes with the virus's replication. But most of us wait longer than that before seeing our physician," Dr. Friedman says.

"Other than that, there's very little you can do except to try and get through it as comfortably as possible."

TUBERCULOSIS (TB)

"Consumption" was once its name, and there were homes all over the country for people who had it—homes called sanitariums.

When the choked lungs and bloody coughing became too much for a family to handle, the lucky ones with money were installed in posh rest homes in places like Arizona and New Mexico. The dry desert air, it was thought, would help the lungs heal.

Tuberculosis is a bacterial infection that can affect any part of the body but usually takes up residence in the lungs. Dry air may have helped some of its early victims, but modern antibiotics have now proved much more effective. In fact, they almost made this killer extinct—until AIDS came along. Now its numbers are climbing again with the help of an immune system wrecker that makes TB carriers—and many of us *carry* the bacteria—suddenly vulnerable to a bug that normally wouldn't make a small dent in their defenses.

"It's a slowly progressing pneumonia," Dr. Friedman says. "Over a period of months, it causes coughs, fever and a general debility, until the typical patient finally sees a doctor. Then it's diagnosed through X-rays."

The primary drug used to combat tuberculosis is called INH, short for isoniazid. It's used alone as a prophylaxis—usually for about a year, after a skin test identifies someone as a carrier who hasn't yet developed the disease. And it's used in combination with other drugs—usually ethambutol and rifampin or pyrazinamide—to battle active cases.

The good news? Modern antibiotics are so effective against the disease that TB is almost never fatal.

STREP THROAT

This nasty little pain in the voice box bites almost everyone at least once before they're old enough to drive. Blame it on the bacteria that give it its name—streptococci, vicious little organisms that can cause tonsillitis, laryngitis or more general fever and swelling. They're also a very common cause of pneumonia in the hospitalized.

"Strep hits children most frequently," Dr. Friedman says. "It usually lasts for a week and then fades."

In fact, more than 250,000 cases were reported to the CDC in a recent year. The actual number is probably much larger, since many cases go unreported. Standard treatment for this infection, which is rarely a serious threat, is penicillin. If left untreated, however, strep throat can lead to rheumatic fever, which causes damage to the lining of the heart.

COMMON COLD

Sniffle, sniffle. Drip, drip. Cough, wheeze. Ahhhhhh-CHO-O-O-O!

It's an ancient tyranny, one we could well live without. But it doesn't seem likely we'll manage to escape the miserable grasp of the common cold anytime in the near future.

"There are many different viruses that cause the common cold," Dr. Friedman says. "Rhinovirus is probably the most common, but there are more than 90 that can produce a cold in the average person."

It's no wonder the cold's so common! If you

didn't get one this year, your chances of getting one next year are very good. But despite the fact that so many people suffer through a cold, there's still very little that can be done about it.

"You can, in fact, develop immunity to a particular cold virus," Dr. Friedman says, "and the immune response probably shortens the course of the infection. But immunity to one virus does not confer protection from any of the others. That's the reason that we get colds again and again."

Treatment? "Not much," Dr. Friedman says. It's *the* classic case where you can ease the symptoms but you can't treat the cause.

"Take something for runny nose and fever, but that's about it," he says. Then just let it run its course.

LEGIONNAIRES' DISEASE

This is *not* something that used to kill large numbers of French Foreign Legionnaires in Algeria. It is a highly fatal bacterial infection, caused by a bug that was first isolated during a lethal outbreak in 1976 at an American Legion convention in Philadelphia.

Legionnaires' disease produces high fever, abdominal pain, headache and pneumonia. It is apparently transmitted most effectively in an aerosol form—in the warm, moist air of the cooling systems of air conditioning systems. As a result, cases usually occur in clusters.

"It's in the water, but you can't get it by drinking," Dr. Friedman says. "Aerosol produced by that water through evaporation, however, may carry the bacteria into your lungs. In Philadelphia, the air-conditioning system may have carried it throughout the hotel involved."

One comforting thought: Legionnaires' disease isn't common. In a recent year, less than a thousand people developed the disease. Erythromycin is the antibiotic of choice.

"It's hard to culture this bacteria, which means it's hard to make a positive diagnosis. So when we suspect that it's the agent involved, we use a drug that's broadly effective instead of the more narrowly active antibiotics," Dr. Friedman explains.

SINUSITIS

Your nose hurts, your eyes hurt, your *eyebrows* hurt. And when you sneeze . . . that much pain can't be good for anyone.

Sinusitis is medicalese for inflammation of the sinuses. A lot of things can cause it, but most go by the name of bacteria.

It generally shows up as pain in and around the sinus cavities, headache, fever and swelling. There's usually a discharge from the nose, too.

Many antibiotics are effective against sinusitis. The choice is your doctor's. They're often prescribed, by the way, in combination with a decongestant to make breathing easier.

LARYNGITIS

What? What was that? Speak up there—we can't hear you.

Losing your voice is probably the best known consequence of laryngitis, although this inflammation of the voice box can produce everything from a bit of gravel in your communications to total absence of your sound-production capability.

Laryngitis is usually caused by a virus—most often a member of the para-influenza family of viruses. "They usually produce sore throat, lost or hoarse voice, mild pain and swelling," Dr. Friedman says. "There's very little we can do about them, but that's not critical, since they're usually very mild infections. Something to keep the fever down is the usual prescription."

TONSILLITIS

This is often the result of a strep infection and can be thought of in the same terms as strep throat. See the strep throat entry on page 161 for treatment recommendations.

DIPHTHERIA

This upper respiratory infection killed large numbers of children in the early years of the century. But the advent of effective vaccines has made it a medical rarity today: A series of shots in the first year of life effectively protects us against this ancient killer.

"Diphtheria is almost never seen as an active infection in this country today," Dr. Friedman says. CDC data agree with him—*one* case was reported in a recent year.

In the unlikely event that someone does develop the disease, it can be treated effectively with antibiotics.

PERTUSSIS

Another ancient enemy, whooping cough is almost a historical footnote—though not quite—because of the miracle of modern vaccines. Only about 2,000 cases were reported in a recent year, though the actual number may be slightly higher.

This bacterial infection typically inflames the entire respiratory tract, producing large amounts of phlegm and the distinct crowing cough that it's named after. Most common in children, it occurs most frequently in the winter and is extremely contagious. Standard treatment is erythromycin.

"One concern with whooping cough is the vaccine," Dr. Friedman says. "A small number of people may experience an allergic reaction, occasionally resulting in neurological impairment—paralysis, for example. But for the most of us the vaccine is a whole lot safer than the disease."

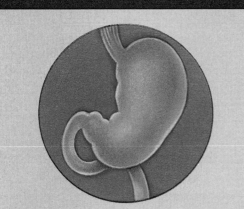

GASTROINTESTINAL INFECTIONS

HEPATITIS

"Gee, Dad, how come you're yellow all over?"

Turning yellow is one of the milder consequences of hepatitis, or inflammation of the liver. Others include mild fever, coma and even death. In a recent year, almost 60,000 cases were reported. Hepatitis is usually broken into several separate categories.

Type A, or infectious hepatitis, is caused by a virus that can be transmitted through food or liquids. It does not cause permanent liver damage in most cases, and recovery is usually complete.

Poor sanitation is the major cause of infectious hepatitis for most people—chiefly in the Third World—where water supplies are often contaminated. Injections of immunoglobulin (human antibody) confer effective but short-term protection against infection for travelers.

Type B, or serum hepatitis, is more insidious than type A. There's a long incubation period for the virus before symptoms develop, and it's at this time that the disease is most contagious. It's most commonly spread by contaminated needles or blood transfusions.

Hepatitis B can resolve itself in short order or develop into chronic liver disease that can go on for years. No specific therapy is available at the present time, though medical personnel and other high-risk groups may be vaccinated to protect against the disease.

Non-A/Non-B hepatitis is the third type. "Essentially, this means that the symptoms of hepatitis are present, the doctor asks for tests, and they come back negative for type A and type B," says Dr. Friedman. "There's some *other* infectious agent at work that closely resembles B, but we can't detect it at this time."

Liver function tests can, however, exclude about half of those blood donors who do carry that unknown infectious agent.

SHIGELLOSIS

Named after the bacteria that causes it—shigella—this is a very severe but short-lived dysentery. Symptoms include bad diarrhea and fever. It's relatively common—more than 17,000 cases were reported to the CDC in a recent year. But it's rarely life-threatening.

"Shigellosis can be treated with a number of antibiotics," Dr. Friedman says, "but often—cultures are required for diagnosis—the patient's better by the time you get the test results back."

In this country, the disease is usually the result of eating contaminated shellfish, though it's also transmitted by direct contact—a handshake, for example, with an infected person or via fecal material in the water supply. Ampicillin is a frequently used antibiotic.

TYPHOID

Indiana Jones might come down with this in the course of his peregrinations about the world's darkest jungles and most remote film sets. But you're not likely to: Less than 400 cases were reported in the United States in a recent year.

Typhoid is an infection generated by a strain of salmonella bacteria. Common symptoms include muscle aches, diarrhea, fever, a rash, enlargement of the spleen, chills and abdominal swelling.

"A person with typhoid is very ill," Dr. Friedman says. "It's a serious disease that left untreated will often kill the patient. But with proper care, it's not usually fatal."

Transmitted in fecal material, typhoid is almost always acquired by drinking contaminated water or having physical contact with a victim. Chloramphenicol is the drug of choice.

CHOLERA

The popular image of cholera as a rampaging killer may be more a product of the shortage of medical facilities in its chief stomping grounds—the Third World—than the power of the disease itself.

"A toxin released by the bacteria responsible causes the severe dysentery [diarrhea] that characterizes this disease," Dr. Friedman says. "The illness only lasts three or four days, and dehydration is the major threat. So if you can replace the fluid lost—by mouth, or, when necessary, with an IV—there's no problem."

Tetracycline is often used to shorten the term of the disease, but most Americans won't ever learn that: In this nation, the most common cause of cholera is eating contaminated shellfish (the bacteria is endemic in Southeastern waters), but in a recent year only *one* U.S. resident came down with cholera.

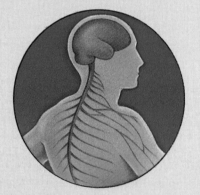

NERVOUS SYSTEM INFECTIONS

MENINGITIS

"Mind on fire" is not a bad way to think of this disease's effect, when bacterial or viral invasion generates swelling and inflammation of the diaphanous layer of tissue covering the brain.

"A lot of viruses and a lot of bacteria can cause meningitis, but there's an important difference between the two," Dr. Friedman says. "Viral meningitis tends to be a very mild disease, while the bacterial form can be very, very serious—in fact, fatal."

Common symptoms are violent headaches, vomiting, fever and the prime distinguishing characteristic: a stiff neck. (Moving the neck stretches the meningal membrane, causing pain.)

Meningococcal bacteria are the chief source of bacterial meningitis, which is highly contagious: Coughing and contact both spread it. Patients are usually isolated until they've been under treatment for at least 24 hours.

A group of organisms called enteroviruses is the most common cause of the aseptic, or noninfectious, form of viral meningitis, which frequently strikes children in the summer months. Mumps and polio virus are two leading causes of the infectious viral forms.

Treatment varies: When a virus is involved, there's not much the doctor can do except try to make the patient comfortable. When bacterial causes are suspected, broad-spectrum antibiotics are used in combination until the specific organism is identified.

ENCEPHALITIS

Sometimes called sleeping sickness, victims of this disease slip into a deep lethargy that in reality bears little resemblance to rest.

Encephalitis is actually a life-threatening inflammation of the brain that is usually the result of viral infection.

"The virus that is probably the most severe and

the most common is herpes simplex—the same one that causes genital herpes and cold sores—but the list of viruses that *can* cause it is a long one," Dr. Friedman says.

Symptoms are similar to those of meningitis—fever, vomiting, headaches and occasionally convulsions. But encephalitis usually causes some sort of mental dysfunction also, which tells the physician that the brain itself is involved. More than 1,000 cases were reported to the CDC in a recent year.

"We can treat it with acyclovir if herpes is the cause, but there's very little we can do otherwise," Dr. Friedman says.

What happens if you get it? The answer isn't reassuring. The majority of patients survive, but a "significant" number die, Dr. Friedman says.

TETANUS

Lockjaw, it's called—and that's exactly what happens when the *Clostridium tetani* bacteria injected into your body when you step on that rusty nail start releasing their neurotoxins.

The results include trismus—lockjaw itself—muscle spasms and seizures.

"Penicillin is an effective treatment, but the main emphasis today is prophylactic—a vaccination that all of us get with our whooping cough and diphtheria shots," Dr. Friedman says.

It must be working. In a recent year, the CDC reported a grand total of only 74 cases.

POLIO

A killer disease that once ravaged the nation with relative impunity, polio didn't distinguish between the lofty and the lowly: President Franklin Delano Roosevelt wore braces as the result of his brush with the virus.

But times have changed.

"Polio is now extremely rare in this country, courtesy of very good vaccines," Dr. Friedman says. In fact, only eight cases were reported to the CDC in a recent year.

Transmission usually occurs through direct contact with an infected person or with contaminated materials. Common symptoms are headache, fever and paralysis of an arm, leg or occasionally the face. Death can occur if the respiratory muscles are involved.

Prevention—by means of vaccination—is the preferred treatment, since very little can be done to combat the disease itself once infection occurs.

BOTULISM

The good old days weren't so good in some ways. When *everyone* did their own canning, a lot more people came down with this particularly vicious form of food poisoning.

Botulism is one possible—and very deadly—consequence of canning foods improperly. Those Americans still canning are apparently doing so with care, since only 123 cases were reported to the CDC in a recent year.

Typical symptoms include vomiting, abdominal pain and difficulty breathing, all caused by a neurotoxin released by the killer bacteria.

"When deaths have occurred from botulism, they've usually been the result of respiratory difficulties," Dr. Friedman says.

OTITIS MEDIA

Any parent with small children should be familiar with the cry: "Mommy, my ear hurts! Make it stop!" Otitis means inflammation of the ear, and it's almost always the result of bacterial infection. It affects the middle ear, just behind the eardrum, and tends to limit its assaults to children.

"An opening at the back of the throat that normally drains that area gets plugged, allowing the bacteria to build up," Dr. Friedman says.

Common symptoms include earache and fever. If left untreated, which rarely happens in the United States, a punctured eardrum can result—with permanent loss of hearing the consequence. In severe cases, a tube may be inserted by the doctor to drain the infection, but antibiotics like cefaclor usually do the job.

GERMAN MEASLES (RUBELLA)

This is a mild viral infection that produces a distinguishing red rash—first on the head and scalp, then on the arms and body. Less than 1,000 cases were reported to the CDC in a recent year, making it one of the more rare infections on this list.

Most children and adults who get rubella survive unscathed with normal support therapy: fluids and something for fever. It's not very severe—most people experience only mild fever, sore throat and a stiff neck. And it typically runs its course in almost no time—two to three days. But pregnant women should avoid it at all costs.

"That's the chief concern with this disease," Dr. Friedman says. "It can produce significant abnormalities in the unborn child."

What abnormalities it produces depends in large part on when it occurs during pregnancy. But the list includes heart defects, cataracts, mental retardation and deafness.

Prevention is chiefly a matter of avoiding contact with people who have rubella, since it's spread chiefly through contact and coughing. But a vaccine is available that is usually given to children in their second year. The vaccine or the infection both confer lifetime immunity.

MEASLES

Red spots all over the face, and mothers chanting, "Don't scratch, don't scratch." That's measles for most of us.

But measles isn't harmless. Less than 3,000 people came down with it in a recent year, but if you were one of them, you were much sicker than someone else who came down with the German version. In fact, you were wrestling with a potentially life-threatening illness.

"Measles can migrate to the brain and produce encephalitis," Dr. Friedman says. "That makes it something you can't afford to take lightly—a viral brain infection can easily kill." The reassuring news is that it happens to only ¹⁄₁₀ of 1 percent of all of us (or 3 out of 3,000).

Measles most often occur in midwinter or spring, following two or three cycles. Cases typically occur in clusters—mild epidemics that grow through contact with infected people or things they've touched.

You know you've got the disease if you've been tired and uncomfortable for a couple of days— maybe running a slight fever, too, with a runny nose and cough—and then all of a sudden this rash starts crawling down your body from your hairline.

Thirty-six hours later the rash is so ugly you'd scare Godzilla: You're blanketed in ¼-inch pink spots that itch like crazy, as well as large red blotches.

But again, there's good news to temper the bad. The rash usually disappears after three or four days. Antihistamines temper the itching. And

since children are now regularly vaccinated against measles on or about their fifteenth month, the disease should become even rarer.

Treatment recommendations: rest, fluids and medication for relief of symptoms, including calamine lotion or antihistamines for itching.

MUMPS

"Gosh, Mom, my neck sure hurts."

That's all mumps is for most of us—a childhood memory of a sore neck wrapped in the blankets mothers seemed to think were medical necessities back then.

This classic childhood infection causes swelling of the salivary glands, producing the typical puffy neck. A viral infection, it's somewhat less dangerous than measles, and a good vaccine is available. But Dr. Friedman nonetheless cautions against taking it lightly: "Just like measles, it can migrate to the brain and cause encephalitis that could be fatal."

About 3,000 people—mostly children, of course—came down with mumps in a recent year. And the chances of having it turn serious are very, very small.

RABIES

Only three human cases were reported in a recent year, but this potentially lethal virus is alive and well in animal populations, and it may be increasing.

"We see very, very little rabies today," Dr. Friedman says. "Unless you're bitten by a rabid animal, your chances of getting it are almost nonexistent."

Dogs and cats are almost never rabid, Dr. Friedman says, thanks to an extremely effective vaccination program. Raccoons are common culprits, however, as well as other wild animals that coexist well with human settlement.

But even if you're bitten by a potentially rabid animal, you're almost certainly not going to develop the disease itself. An excellent vaccine is available that stops the disease in its tracks—or rather, tricks your immune system into stomping it dead.

The catch: You can't wait for a positive diagnosis to start treatment.

"You really need to start the injections within 48 hours of possible infection," Dr. Friedman says. The good news: Despite popular myth, you get the five shots in your arm, not your stomach.

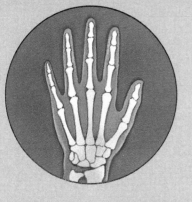

BONE, JOINT AND SKIN INFECTIONS

CHICKEN POX

Small, itchy blisters in awkward places that no normal human being could possibly scratch—chicken pox is a nearly universal childhood experience.

This normally mild viral infection produces sore throat, fever and a distinctive rash of small pustules covering the whole body, but it's not much of threat to most people.

"Unless the individual has a compromised immune system (a child with leukemia, for example), it's really a rather mild infection that most come through without damage," Dr. Friedman says.

If you had chicken pox as a child, you're unlikely to get it again. But it *can* recur in adulthood. It may produce the same symptoms it does in children, but it occasionally metamorphoses into something called shingles—a painful infection of the nerves. Shingles is relatively rare before age 50.

Treatment for chicken pox is limited to antivirals like acyclovir (Zovirax) and medication for relief of symptoms.

SEPTIC ARTHRITIS

A joint infection, usually of bacterial origin, this bears no relation to rheumatoid and other common forms of arthritis, which develop for entirely different reasons.

Staphylococcus aureus is a common cause, but septic arthritis can also be a consequence of untreated gonorrhea. Symptoms include pain, swelling in the joint and fever. Tissue damage often results in loss of motion in the infected joint.

Definitive diagnosis is made by sampling fluid from the joint. Treatment varies with the cause: penicillin if gonococcal bacteria are responsible, cephalosporins or similar antibiotics if it's staph.

OSTEOMYELITIS

This is an infection of the bone, caused by bacteria. In children, the disease may develop from an initial skin infection. But the bug can also start its journey from a sore throat or migrate to the bone after a cut or other wound provides a port of entry.

In adults, osteomyelitis is usually associated with some kind of major trauma—a broken leg where the bone sticks out, for example. Staphylococcus is a commonly involved bacteria. Treatment requires taking antibiotics for up to six weeks. Often, surgery is necessary to remove the infected tissue.

FURUNCLES AND CARBUNCLES

Furuncle is simply another name for the infamous boil—a pus-filled blister that can occur just about anywhere on the body.

Carbuncles are boils on parade—blister clusters instead of single boils. Both are the result of infection with *Staphylococcus aureus*. Carbuncles are commonly associated with poor health. They develop when disease or poor nutrition compromises the immune system's ability to suppress the staph bacteria that normally exists on your skin.

Treatment consists of appropriate antibiotics—oxycillin, for example—and lancing to drain individual boils.

TOXIC SHOCK SYNDROME (TSS)

TSS was initially a mystery disease of the worst kind—no one knew what it was or how it killed people.

But rest easy. Most of the answers are now in. TSS is apparently the result of exposure to toxins produced in the vagina by *Staphylococcus aureus*—and it might legitimately be called *tampon* shock syndrome.

Under certain circumstances, high-absorbency tampons apparently cause TSS by creating an environment in the vagina where much-higher-than-normal levels of bacteria can accumulate. But the precise mechanism isn't known.

Typical symptoms of this life-threatening illness include high fever, vomiting, diarrhea and muscle aches. Antibiotics work against the bacteria, but victims may die if medical support appropriate to shock—plasma, to maintain blood volume, and general fluid replacement—is not available. The numbers, however, are comforting: Only 482 cases were reported in a recent year.

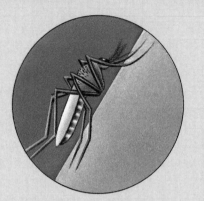

INSECT-BORNE INFECTIONS

ROCKY MOUNTAIN SPOTTED FEVER

Chiefly a summer phenomenon, this is a bacterial infection transmitted by ticks. Campers and hikers are at most risk for obvious reasons, but ticks carried into the house by your dog can also transmit the disease—to you, not the pooch. Less than 1,000 cases were reported in a recent year, making your chances of getting it small indeed. But just in case, typical symptoms include a rash—the spots—muscle aches and fever. Don't take this disease lightly if you do get it. It can kill, Dr. Friedman says. But antibiotics like chloramphenicol are very effective in reversing the infection.

LYME ARTHRITIS

Named after the Connecticut town where it was discovered, this is an infection that typically takes up residence in large joints like the shoulders, knees and elbows. Symptoms include pain, swelling and muscle aches. The disease is transmitted by tick bites.

A characteristic rash—flushed red patches of skin that enlarge slowly while the center clears—usually appears several weeks after infection and is a sure indicator that this is not normal arthritis you're dealing with.

And that's good news. Lyme's no more lethal than other forms of arthritis, but it's distinctly more curable: Treatment with tetracyline or penicillin whips the bug, and with it the arthritis.

MALARIA

This is probably the one disease everyone thinks of when they think of mosquitoes. Unlike others on this list, it's not caused by a virus or species of bacteria. A *parasite* is responsible: *Plasmodium malariae,* to be exact. Each new generation of protozoa growing in the body (and eating your red blood cells, incidentally) generates a new round of the fever, sweating and chills associated with the infection.

Only about a thousand Americans came down with malaria in a recent year, but it continues to affect large numbers in the Third World. Chloroquine phosphate is the antibiotic of choice, although the old standby quinine may be called in to battle resistant strains occasionally found in Southeast Asia, South America and parts of Africa.

TULAREMIA

Rabbit fever to some folks, tularemia is named after the town where it was first characterized—Tulare, California. A bacterial infection resembling plague—it also makes the lymph glands beneath the arms swell and, like plague, it's carried by rodents—tularemia is transmitted by ticks, fleas and deerflies. It causes fever, chills, muscle aches and headaches. Infection often occurs in hunters who skin infected animals with their bare hands, thus exposing themselves to fleas or contaminated blood. But infection is rare—less than 300 cases were reported in a recent year—and two drugs (streptomycin and tetracycline) effectively stop the responsible bacteria.

SOURCES & CREDITS

SOURCE NOTES

Children

page 15

"When to Immunize," compiled with information supplied by the American Academy of Pediatrics.

Home

page 44

"Detoxify Your Household Cleaners," adapted from "Safe at Home?" by Linda Hunter, *Rodale's Practical Homeowner*, October 1986.

Hospitals

page 48

"Where Germs Get an Education," adapted from "Nosocomial Infection Surveillance 1984," by Teresa C. Horan, M.P.H., et al., *CDC Surveillance Summaries*, vol. 35, no. 1ss.

Medications

pages 76–77

"Medications That Help the Immune System," compiled by Terry Phillips, Ph.D., director of Immunogenetics and Immunochemistry Laboratories, George Washington University Medical Center, Washington, D.C.

Self-Care for Everyday Infections

page 129

"Fever: Danger Rises with Age," adapted from "Effects of Aging on Fever," *The Journal of the American Geriatrics Society*, April 1984.

page 134

"Lysine Helps Herpes Sufferers," adapted from "Success of L-Lysine Therapy in Frequently Recurrent Herpes Simplex Infection," by Richard S. Griffith et. al., *Dermatologica*, vol. 175, 1987.

page 135

"Wound Healing Rates of First-Aid Products," adapted from "Comparison of Topical Antibiotics, Ointments, a Wound Protectant and Antiseptics for the Treatment of Human Blister Wounds Contaminated with *Staphylococcus aureus*," by James Leyden, M.D., and Nora M. Bartelt. *Journal of Family Practice*, vol. 24, no. 6, 1987.

Smoking

page 148

"Leukocytes on the March" adapted from "The Leukocyte Count," by Diana B. Petitti and Harold Kipp, *American Journal of Epidemiology*, January 1986.

page 149

"Cigarettes Cripple Cilia," adapted from *Tobacco and Your Health*, by Harold S. Diehl, M.D. (New York: McGraw-Hill Book Company, 1969).

PHOTOGRAPHY CREDITS

Cover: Angelo M. Caggiano

Staff Photographers: Angelo M. Caggiano: pp. 9; 30. Carl Doney: p. 132. Donna

M. Hornberger: pp. 121; 124. Ed Landrock: pp. 88–89, top. Alison Miksch: p. 45. Christie C. Tito: pp. 10-11; 15; 24; 32, top; 36; 47; 49; 90–91; 92; 93; 94; 96; 97; 98; 99; 100–101; 107; 120; 125; 138. Sally Shenk Ullman: pp. 7, left; 12; 32-33, bottom; 136.

Other Photographers: All Sport/Vandystadt: p. 29. AP/Wide World Photos: p. 65. John Auel/Leo de Wys, Inc.: p. 55. Paul Barton/The Stock Market: p. 95. David Brownell: pp. 6, right; 26-27. Kathleen Thormod Carr/Leo de Wys, Inc.: p. 88, bottom. Comstock: p. 85. Alan Dolgin/Leo de Wys, Inc.: p. 108. Jack Fields/Photo Researchers, Inc.: p. 20. Chuck Fishman: p. 83. Chuck Fishman/Woodfin Camp: p. 39. Gamma-Liaison: p. 72. E. D. Getzoff and J. A. Tainer/Scripps Clinic: p. 69. Hans Huber Medical Publishers, Bern, Switzerland: p. 80. J. Heibeler/Leo de Wys, Inc.: p. 153. Brian King/Leo de Wys, Inc.: p. 71. R. Lopez/FPG International: p. 154. Mr. Mookerjee, from *Yantra: The Tantric Symbol of Cosmic Unity* by Madhu Khanna, Plate 62, p. 113 (Thames and Hudson): p. 87. David Muench: p. 103. Michael Neveux: p. 75. Dr. Lennart Nilsson copyright Boehringer Ingelheim International GmbH: p. 143. Dr. Lennart Nilsson copyright Boehringer Ingelheim International GmbH, from *The Body Victorious:* pp. 7, right; 50-51; 54; 57; 59; 60; 62-63. Phototeque: p. 21.

Jim Pickerell/FPG International: p. 81. H. Armstrong Roberts/Zesa: p. 102. Fred L. Saracino: p. 105. Sue Shea/Photo Researchers, Inc.: p. 106. Mark Sherman/Bruce Coleman, Inc.: p. 111. Shostal Associates: pp. 118-19. Steinhart Aquarium/Photo Researchers, Inc.: p. 141. Dova Wilson/Westock: p. 89, bottom. Tom Zimberoff/Sygma: pp. 66-67, top.

Additional Photographs Courtesy of: Bellevue Stratford Hotel: p. 65. Centers for Disease Control: pp. 6, left; 64; 67, bottom. NASA: p. 157. National Archive: p. 115. National Library of Medicine: p. 112. World Health Organization: p. 147.

Photographic Stylists: Marianne G. Laubach: pp. 90–91; 92; 93; 94; 96; 97; 98; 99; 100–101. Kay Seng Lichthardt: pp. 32-33, bottom. Pamela Simpson: pp. 10-11; 30; 125.

ILLUSTRATION CREDITS

Laura Cornell: pp. 35; 40; 130; 150. Mellisa Edmonds: pp. 11; 23; 25; 28; 31; 33; 37; 46; 104; 109; 110; 113; 122; 123; 126; 128; 133; 145; 151. Kathi Ember: pp. 116; 158; 160; 163; 164; 167; 168. Leslie Flis: pp. 48; 129; 134; 135; 148. Steve Heimann: p. 17. Bradley Keough: p. 18. Narda Lebo: pp. 7; 22; 38; 52-53; 79; 149. Susan Rosenberger: pp. 42-43; 131. Wallop: p. 152.

INDEX

Note: Page references in **boldface** indicate tables. References in *italic* indicate illustrations.

beta-carotene and, 92
cocaine and, 21
immunity and, 62–63
killer cells and, 56, *57*, 58
mind and, 78, 80, *80*, 81
personality type and, 81
selenium and, 98–99
viruses linked to, 66
vitamin A and, 90
vitamin E and, 96
Candida, 140, 160
Candida albicans, 92
Canine distemper, 108
Canine parvovirus, 108
Canker sores, 122–23
Capsaicin, 136
Carbuncles, 167
Cats, 107, 110–11
CDC. *See* Centers for Disease Control (CDC), infection fighting at
Cefaclor, 165
Ceftriaxone, 159
Cellar, microbes in, 41, *42*, 44
Cells. *See* Immune system, mechanism of *and specific types*
Centers for Disease Control (CDC), infection fighting at, 64–67
Central nervous system infections, 23, 164–66
Cephalosporins, 75, **76**, 167
Cervical cancer, herpes and, 135
Chagas disease, 118–19
Chicken pox, 13, 14, 15, **15**, 136, 167
Children
        immunity and, 10–15
        nursery disinfection for, *42*, 44–45
        pets and, 107
        respiratory infections in, 162, 163
Chlamydia, 16, 142, 145, 159–60
Chloramphenicol, **76**, 164, 168
Chloroquine phosphate, 168
Cholera, 153, 164
Cigarette smoking, 148–49
Cilia, smoking and, 149
Cirrhosis, alcoholic, 25

Cleaners, household, toxicity of, **44**
Clostridium botulinum, 35, 37
Clostridium tetani, 165
Clotrimazole, 160
Cocaine, 20–21
Cognitive structuring, 84
Colds, 161–62
        in children, 10–11
        drugs to prevent, 73
        self-care for, 124–27
Cold sores, self-care for, 123–24
Colorado tick fever, 119
Complement, 52, 60
Condoms, 134, 144, 145
Congenital ichthyosiform erythroderma, 78
Conjunctivitis, 25
        self-care for, 127
Cooking, 34
Copper, 99–100
Corticosteroids, 74, 79
Cough
        in children, 11, 13, 14
        as sign of serious infection, 24
        from smoking, 149
        whooping, 13, 15, **15**, 162–63
Crystallography, 3-D, *69*, 72
Cuts, self-care for, 135–37
Cyclosporine, 74
Cystic fibrosis, 70
Cystic hydatid disease, 119
Cystitis, self-care for, 127–28

D

Dehydration, from fever, 129
Dermacentor andersoni, 119
Diabetes, 23, 70
Diarrhea, 102, 150–51
Diet. *See also* Nutrition
        cystitis and, 127, 128
Diphtheria, 15, **15**, 162
DNA, 19, 68, *69*
Docosahexaenoic acid (DHA), 100
Dogs, 107–9
DPT (diphtheria, pertussis, tetanus) vaccine, 13, **15**
Driving, influenza and, 130

Drugs
        to fight viruses, 71–73
        immune system and, 20–21, 74–75, **76–77**
Dust, 45

E

E. coli. See Escherichia coli
Earaches, 25
Ear infections, 23
        in children, 11–12, 75, 165
Ebola-Marburg virus, 67
Eicosapentaenoic acid (EPA), 100, 101
Elderly. *See also* Aging
        fever in, 129
        influenza in, 131
        vitamin B$_6$ and, 93
        zinc and, 98
Elephantiasis, 118
ELISA. *See* Enzyme-linked immunosorbent assay
Emergency infections, 22–25
Emotions, immunity and, 78–87
Encephalitis, 23, 164–65, 166
        in children, 13
        in northern countries, 119
Endorphins, 84
Enteroviruses, 164
Enzyme-linked immunosorbent assay (ELISA), 19
Epidemic Intelligence Service (EIS), 64–65
Epidemics, 113–14
Epidemiology, studied by CDC, 64–67
Epiglottiditis, in children, 13
Epinephrine, 79
Epstein-Barr virus, 16, 19
Erythroderma, congenital ichthyosiform, 78
Erythromycin, 162, 163
Escherichia coli, *54*, 150–51
Ethambutol, 161
E$_2$, 96, 100
Exercise, 26–32
        effect of, 27–28